Midlife
Journeys

Midlife Journeys

A TRAVELER'S GUIDE

Richard P. Olson

THE PILGRIM PRESS
Cleveland, Ohio

The Pilgrim Press, Cleveland, Ohio 44115

© 1996 by Richard P. Olson

Grateful acknowledgment to Judson Press for permission to reprint material from *Midlife: A Time to Discover, A Time to Decide*, by Richard P. Olson. "The Veteran" by Dorothy Parker, copyright 1926, renewed 1954 by Dorothy Parker, from *The Portable Dorothy Parker* by Dorothy Parker, introduction by Brendan Gill. Used by permission of Viking Penguin, a division of Penguin Books USA Inc.

Biblical quotations are from the New Revised Standard Version of the Bible, © 1989 by the Division of Christian Education of the National Council of the Churches of Christ in the U.S.A., and are used by permission

01 00 99 98 97 96   5 4 3 2 1

Library of Congress Cataloging-in-Publication Data
Olson, Richard P.
    Midlife journeys : a traveler's guide / Richard P. Olson.
        p.   cm.
    Includes bibliographical references and index.
    ISBN 0-8298-1142-7 (alk. paper)
        1. Life change events—Religious aspects—Christianity.
    2. Midlife crisis—Religious aspects—Christianity.   3. Adjustment
(Psychology)—Religious aspects—Christianity.   4. Olson, Richard P.
I. Title.
BV4509.5047   1996
248.8'4—dc20
                                                        96-30146
                                                             CIP

Contents

I

Midlife
in Broad
Perspective

Introduction

A Personal Reflection on the Midlife Journey

I DON'T KNOW EXACTLY why, but I have always been fascinated with adult growth and development—both others' and my own. Birthdays seem to symbolize this process for me. Let me tell you about four of my adult birthdays. As I do this, I invite you to reflect on key moments in your midlife years as well.

I was puzzled by feelings of sadness and confusion that surrounded me at the time of my thirty-third birthday. It was hard to know why. I thought that I was where I wanted to be, doing what I wanted to do. I had finished (for a time) a good education. Mary Ann and I had been married for ten years. We were parents of three daughters, ages seven, five, and two. I was practicing the profession I thought I wanted to do, pastoral ministry, and seemed to be doing it competently. But there were questions in my mind about career. Did I want to keep doing this? Or would I make a better contribution and feel more at home in an academic career? Should I go back and get the credentials to do that?

When that thirty-third birthday came, I was aware of restlessness and upset for which I could not account. Not sure what to do with these feelings, I confided them to Dave and Mary.

Dave and Mary were close friends and members of my congregation. He was director of social services at a nearby progressive, medium-security prison, and she was a nurse. In his early thirties, Dave had suffered a much more severe crisis—a massive, life-threatening heart attack. Now partially recovered, he was back at work full-time.

In response to this health crisis and continuing uncertainty, Dave and Mary had developed a deep appreciation for each day. They lived life with a zest that was expressed in, among other things, Dave's zany sense of humor. Dave had a stuttering handicap, which often heightened the anticipation of his one-liners.

"I don't know why I'm so upset about being thirty-three," I told them. "I guess it's that I am halfway to retirement and it doesn't feel like I've accomplished much."

"That's not it, Dick," Dave responded. "You're just upset that you haven't got yourself crucified yet!"

Whatever the reasons, my family and I made some drastic changes on my behalf shortly after that thirty-third birthday. We resigned that pastorate and traveled halfway across the country. There I accepted another pastoral position, where I could also pursue doctoral studies and widen our options.

With the passage of time, I completed the doctorate and intended to change careers. I didn't find a job in the academic field, however, so I returned to another pastorate in the Midwest.

Then came my fortieth birthday. I had all but forgotten that unease around my thirty-third. However, the pain of that earlier birthday was minor compared to what hit me on the fortieth.

I was shocked at my response. Someone once said that on your fortieth birthday you become ten years older, and I felt it. It became clear why Jack Benny got so much laugh mileage out of being "thirty-nine." He did so because turning forty rubs a universal raw nerve—a nerve that was being painfully rubbed within me!

There were several sources of pain at age forty. One was career disappointment. After going to all the work of the doctorate, I was hurt that no career reward came my way. Earlier, when I lost out on an opportunity, I would tell myself, "Oh well, some day." From age forty on, after a turn-down it felt like "never."

Another was concern about my body and my health. I had always enjoyed vigorous health. I had assumed I could do more than others because I needed less sleep. Now things seemed to change. Did I tire more easily? Need more sleep? Have less endurance for a vigorous physical game? Ache more after strenuous exercise? It seemed so. Was that flutter in my chest the early warning of a heart attack, so common to us middle-aged men? After all, a heart attack had killed my father at a relatively young age!

I still don't know whether those physical changes were as severe as they seemed. Maybe in my depression I was imagining things. However, one incident did indeed make clear that my body was changing. My eye examination revealed the need for bifocals. I took the prescription with this disappointing news to my optician, a friend older than I. He looked at the prescription, smiled, and asked, "How old are you, Dick?" "Forty-two," I replied. "You're right on schedule!" he told me.

By far the most troubling themes for me were *time* (or, more accurately, the lack of and shortness of time) and *death*. For several months after my fortieth birthday, death was a daily concern. Either I dreamt about death every night, or the first thought that occurred to me on waking was, "It's too bad about death." Gradually the dreams decreased, but the dread remained. This preoccupation was particularly troubling to me, since I thought I had claimed the Christian faith's perspective on death. I had comforted many people with that very gospel. But what I had offered to others, I seemingly had not adequately grasped for myself.

Martin Luther once said that all of us must do our own believing and our own dying, and now I was discovering the truth of what he said. Quite often, I was called on to minister to persons who were dying. Therefore, I could not entirely ignore or repress the subject of death, as many midlifers do.

Time was closing in on me. I felt that one normal lifetime would not be adequate to achieve my aspirations. My weekly schedule allowed precious few moments to find enjoyment or fulfillment. Part of this was the result of my workaholic lifestyle. That lifestyle no longer made much sense to me, but I was not strong enough or wise enough to change it. Self-pity or resentment over time demands occurred frequently.

There was a sexual component in this midlife turmoil as well—unsettling, but not entirely unpleasant. I had never considered myself particularly attractive to persons of the opposite sex. Rather, to my woman friends I had most often been like a brother—kind, reassuring, comfortable, nonthreatening. But in this midlife turmoil, something changed. Unfamiliar feelings of attraction, romance, sexuality seemed to stir within me and communicate to some women I met. Either I received more such messages at that time or I was more sensitive to them. It was like being an adolescent all over again—only more so. And here I was, a husband, a father, a respected community leader.

Coupled with all this was a feeling that this life passage was absolutely unique, unlike anything before it in my experience. There was also the sense that I was utterly alone in it.

I was fortunate about one thing. As midlife struggles go, mine was relatively mild. I don't think I missed a day of work as a result of it (that Puritan work ethic again). However, I found little joy in what I was doing. I survived, even though the secret inner pain was sometimes nearly overwhelming.

I was fortunate to find some ways to deal with this crisis—ways that I will describe later in this introduction. The worst of it passed. Once I was past the pain, I became fascinated with adult life stages. As a result, I spoke about midlife and sometimes led seminars on it. I also wrote a book on the issue that was rather well received.

During this recovery stage, an opportunity came to visit my friends Dave and Mary. When I was about to leave their house, Dave walked me out to my car. I had been giving one of my daughters driving lessons in this particular car. One day she had playfully plastered the back windows with decals of colorful rainbows and butterflies. I pointed these out to Dave and asked, "Does this car look as if a teenager is getting ready to take it over?" Dave retorted,

"Either that, or it's owned by a middle-aged man who isn't handling midlife very well!"

I don't know how well, but by then I was handling midlife. A relative stability. The comparative calm felt very good indeed.

And then my fiftieth birthday approached.

My children, knowing how difficult my fortieth had been, were worried. One of them asked me, "Dad, are you going to make as big a fuss over being fifty as you did over being forty?" "Why not," I responded, "if there is another book in it for me!" The fact was that I didn't how I would feel about being fifty, or how I would handle it. Shortly before this birthday, Mary Ann and I received word that we would be grandparents. Mary Ann was excited about the prospect and began buying gifts for the anticipated child. I found it hard to be enthusiastic—to me it felt like a message about growing old!

To my delight, I woke up feeling good on my fiftieth birthday. The day was bright and beautiful, and it matched my inner feelings. I called to mind the greeting sent to someone on the same occasion—"Congratulations on your fiftieth birthday. You have just left the old age of youth and entered the youth of old age." I resolved to claim that greeting.

Rather than thinking about death and the shortness of time, as on my fortieth birthday, I was thinking about life and new opportunity. I resolved that I would start something new in my life on that very birthday, and located some key persons to advise me on steps to take to earn my counseling credentials. On my birthday, I made appointments with these people, and I went to see them later in the week. These conversations made it possible to start on that growth process just a few weeks later, and I gained pastoral counseling credentials after a just few years.

On my fiftieth birthday, and for several days following, family and friends from across the country called with supportive greetings. This added to my good feelings. I was surrounded by a wide circle of love.

Five days later, on a Sunday afternoon, I was out mowing my yard when I heard the phone ring. Since my wife was inside near the phone, I kept on mowing. However, I fully expected to be called to the phone for yet another birthday greeting.

But it was something different. "Dick," Mary Ann called, "come to the phone. It's Debbie, Dave's daughter. Dave just died. She wants to know if you can come to be with them and help with the funeral."

And so I spent the second week after my fiftieth birthday burying my friend and grieving with his children and family. (Dave's wife, Mary, had died of cancer two years before. She had been about fifty.) I also helped them with the difficult decisions of how to live life without him.

The years marched on. Toward the end of another decade, a little incident reminded me of my aging process. I had spent the morning in my office preparing to lead a weekend retreat for a church midlife group. At noon I walked to a nearby sandwich shop for a bite to eat. Aware that I didn't have much cash in my pocket, I ordered a bit more carefully than usual so that I could pay. But then I received more change than I expected. As I looked at my receipt I saw that I had been given my first senior citizen's discount!

Quite recently I celebrated my sixtieth birthday. There were joys and compromises on that special day. I wanted to throw myself a party—rent a large cottage at a popular resort area in central Wisconsin and ask my children and their families to spend a weekend with Mary Ann and me. In a crowded tourist season, no such facility was available, so we gathered at a daughter's home a few hours away. One daughter and son-in-law could not come because my daughter was in the advanced stages of pregnancy with our fourth grandchild. That felt okay—I was full of anticipation and hope for another healthy child. Funny, was it possible I had ever felt empty or old at being a grandpa? What fun those other three were and are! As a gift, my children gave me a plane ticket to go and see the new child when she was born. Life felt good and rich.

To be sure, there were new questions on the horizon—how much longer did I want to continue in my career and my present position? Some contemporaries had already retired and many more were speaking of it. I didn't feel ready for that. I still felt full of creativity and enthusiasm. Yet, there also were long hours, too many night meetings, being tied down when I would like to be with family for special occasions. Further, there were changes and needed adjustments in my profession that I found difficult to make. Occasionally I could see the end of this career as I have known it. What lies beyond has not yet come into focus.

So far I have told you an intensely personal story. Others might experience the passing of years quite differently. I do not expect that my personal experiences will be shared by all. There is a great diversity in the ways people experience the passing of years and in the midlife experience itself.

My wife, Mary Ann, for example, might tell the story of her passage through these years in a manner quite unlike my experience. This is not only because she is female and I am male. We are also quite different persons who think, focus, and process things quite differently. She has not had any of the traumas I had around the birthdays mentioned. (This story will be much briefer. This is not because Mary Ann is less important; it is because she is less interested in these subjects and pays less attention to them.)

I remember her fortieth birthday particularly well. Mary Ann is a few years younger than I. She came to this milestone after I had gone through the worst part of my fortieth-birthday crisis. From my struggles and experiences, I was interested to know what she was experiencing.

"How does it feel to be forty, Dear?" I asked her. "Nothing special or unusual," she replied. Unsatisfied, I probed on. "Don't you feel time closing in on you?" "No," she responded. "With the children growing older, I feel I am going to have more time to do the things I want. I feel time opening up to me."

Nor did she seem to have any trauma around earlier or later birthdays. She was passing a thirtieth birthday shortly before I worried about my thirty-third. Busy with the care of our children, she didn't give it much notice. And when she came to her fiftieth, others were much more impressed with that time of passage than she. Her story of pilgrimage through these years would not be built around birthdays.

The crises and transitions for her might be uprootedness, and in particular, geographical moves. These transitions disrupt her life. She dreads the separation from friends and family, from discovered and valued services, from work positions where she has done well and advanced. The need to start all over again finding these essentials of life—that is a difficult task indeed. She is a gifted professional in a field that often promotes from inside firms. Likely, she will have difficulty finding challenging new work. This is coupled with the fact that it will be two steps back from where she was. All this may be for her the most difficult transition of all.

At this point, you might reflect on your own story. I'm sure it is fascinating. I hope that as you listen to our narratives, you will focus on and identify your story more clearly.

As I reflect on the discoveries of living, sharing, and reflecting through these decades, a number of truths come clear. For one thing, adults are fascinating people. Their growth, development, and decisions deserve respect, attention, and loving care. Further, this time called "midlife" is much larger than most people realize. Frequently, I fear, so much attention is given to age-forty crises that equally important times are ignored. Midlife is, I am convinced, a time of life that is at least three decades long. It begins at age thirty or thereabouts, when one may question directions and decisions made up to that time. It continues at least through one's fifties, perhaps into one's sixties, up to retirement. *Midlife is the middle third of one's life!*

Further still, persons going through this portion of the life pilgrimage are not alone, even though they often feel that way. There are helpful writings, both on the general topic of life development in adults and on almost every aspect of that development. As baby boomers enter midlife, this attention is growing. There is literature to help us understand ourselves. There are also people around us with whom we can talk, listen, and offer mutual support.

Again, as adults, we can learn to live our lives even more wisely. Helpful information, stimulating perspectives, challenging questions, and supportive conversations with other adults can all contribute to this increased wisdom.

And again, midlife is a faith journey with profound religious dimensions. We will miss crucially important aspects if we are not
aware of this truth. We will want to claim the faith resources we
know, but we should also examine them for their adequacy. While
from time to time I will refer to the resources of the Christian
faith, I hope these pages speak to all who want to know more
about this journey.

So far, I have told you something of my journey and discussed
some of the convictions that I have formed. Before concluding
this chapter, I want to keep my promise to tell you how I coped
with the changes in my life. I also want to offer a brief strategy to
those of you seeking awareness and wisdom in midlife.

Face the life-stage issues you are experiencing. These issues may cause you
discomfort; however, such unease may lead to important discoveries. Ignoring or repressing difficult feelings rarely leads to growth.
In facing such issues, you may also experience moments of great
joy. I have found it so.

Talk with others about your life pilgrimage. Find others who will speak
with you about your life—possibly a group who may become new
friends. Perhaps you will be able to reflect on your life journeys
together with old friends. And converse with those who have written about the subject. This was such a comfort to me. It was so enriching!

Talk also with yourself and with your God. Personal reflection, journaliz-
ing, meditation, and prayer are valuable resources to gain perspective on ourselves and our lives. It is a time to know ourselves better
and to claim the self we discover. Midlife contains an invitation to
us all—the terrors of this part of life encourage us to become the-
ologians and mystics to find the strength to cope.

I have designed this volume to help you with these strategies.
Most of the midlife issues I experienced, or had reported to me,
are raised in this book. I talk about them in the light of my experience and reading. There may be places where you find my comments too brief. At such times, I will point you to others who have
explored the matter under consideration in more detail. After
each chapter, I will offer some beginning questions. However, if

you form a group to discuss these topics, you will probably not run out of questions of your own. I will regularly point to faith resources, and at the conclusion draw these together in a preliminary "theology of midlife."

As our journeys go on, let our conversations begin.

For Personal or Group Reflection and Discussion

1. Which, if any, birthdays felt particularly significant to you? What do you recall about those birthdays?

2. Were there other life events that, for you, signified important endings or beginnings in your life? Tell about them.

3. As you think about your present stage of life, what are the best aspects of it? The most difficult aspects?

1

Other Maps
of the Midlife
Experience

W E WHO ARE in the middle third of life in the
1990s and beyond are fortunate in one regard.
Scholars and members of the helping professions are giving more
attention to adult life stages. As a result, these people have more to
offer us as we deal with the crises and opportunities in our adult
years.

I am grateful for such scholars and their observations. They
helped me understand and make sense out of the story I told in the
Introduction. They also aided me in making helpful connections
with others going through similar transitions. None of these writers' descriptions fit me exactly at every point. However, each of
them illuminated some aspects of my experience so that I understood myself better and became excited about discoveries still to
come. And so now we turn from a personal view to an overview of
the adult journey.

When I say "overview" I make it sound more simple than it really is. There is no universally accepted life-development theory.
In attempting an overview, I will describe a few key contributors
from earlier in this century. Then I will report the most cogent
critiques and the changed circumstances that modify these views.
That is as close as I can take you to an overview of life stages for

adults. Out of this, you will need to construct your own life-development theory.

Some Significant Historical Contributions

Early in this century, Carl Jung offered some important thoughts on midlife, but no systematic understanding. Three other persons are often cited as making germinal contributions to life-stage theory: Erik Erikson published his views in 1950, and Daniel Levinson and Roger Gould reported their findings in the 1970s. Here are some of the important things they said.

ERIK ERIKSON
The Eight Stages of a Life

Before we can look at Erikson's theory of stages, we need to know some of the central assumptions basic to his view. These are some of the more important ones:

1. For each person there is available a range of psychological strengths and resources. However, at the start of life, many of these strengths exist only in potentiality. They will become available as life unfolds.
2. Though there are variations among individuals in timing and intensity, there is a general underlying pattern in this development.
3. With the emergence of each new psychological resource, there comes a critical time for the individual. This is an important moment in one's personal development. The arrival of this newly developing maturing quality raises a significant question, one that challenges a person's current level of self-understanding. Out of this challenge, another self emerges, like a different person.
4. Each of these developmental challenges brings the person into contact with contradictory impulses, which include both positive and negative aspects of personality.[1]
5. The issues raised by each life stage are related to all the others.
6. None of these life-stage conflicts is resolved once and for all. Unresolved issues may crop up later in life. Indeed, some that seemed fairly well resolved earlier may well reappear later.

7. Personality is formed and shaped by the manner in which the crises caused by dealing with these emerging gifts are managed.[2]

If these assumptions are anywhere near the truth, this is a theory that deserves our careful attention.

Erik Erikson claimed that there are eight stages in the life cycle of a person. The first four of these occur during infancy and childhood:

1. *Infancy: trust versus mistrust.* During this period a person's task is to develop a basic sense of trust in oneself, in others, and in the environment. This comes primarily through the quality of care received in those years.
2. *Early childhood: autonomy versus shame and doubt.* As the child grows, he or she experiments with holding on and letting go. In short, the development of autonomous will occurs during this stage. The task is to learn to use this will without shame and doubt.
3. *Play age: initiative versus guilt.* The child is able to move about freely, communicate, express curiosity, and have fantasies. The child also begins to experience conscience. A youngster begins to discover that it is OK to explore one's outer world and to master aspects of it.
4. *School age: industry versus inferiority.* The child learns how to do and make things with others. One either receives recognition and encouragement in these efforts or experiences a sense of inferiority if the recognition does not come.

Erikson observes that after these four childhood stages, four additional stages occur in the youth and adult years.

5. *Adolescence: identity versus role confusion.* As the person experiences rapid body growth, maturing sexuality, and a gradual approach to adult responsibilities, the task is to integrate these new experiences into a new identity. This new identity has continuity with the identity one felt as a child, but it also has elements of newness and becoming. However, unless the old identity and the new identity are fully integrated (and many pitfalls can occur here), one is not ready for the next stages of life.

6. *Young adulthood: intimacy versus isolation.* As one becomes more secure in one's own identity, the next task is to establish intimacy with one's inner self and with others, both in friendships and in a love-based, mutually satisfying sexual relationship.

7. *Adulthood: generativity versus stagnation.* When one has been able to establish intimacies in adulthood, the next issue is *generativity,* that is, the mature person's interest in establishing and guiding the next generation. This comes with a commitment to caring about the next generation. The person unable to do this may experience a sense of stagnation and impoverishment both within the self and in relationships. (I experience this issue as a powerful truth. In my late midlife, I have a passion for generativity in the form of being available as a mentor. I particularly enjoy teaching, guiding, counseling, encouraging, and supporting younger colleagues in my profession.)

8. *Later adulthood: ego integrity versus despair.* The task is to reach the end of life with ego integrity—acceptance of responsibility for one's life and belief that one's life has had meaning and purpose. Quite obviously, to fail to achieve this is to fall into despair.[3]

Erikson's was a pioneering perspective, first published in 1950. A reading of his theory might lead one to think that life is more linear, orderly, and sequential than it really is. However that is not Erikson's thrust. Rather, he suggests that adults face key developmental issues throughout life. This leads to an even more basic insight that *growth and development take place over a person's entire lifetime.* If that seems perfectly obvious, we are indebted to Erikson for helping it become so clearly understood.

Erikson's overview of life development continues to stimulate study, research, and treatment of adults. Gwen A. Hawley has developed a test instrument by which one may discover one's resolved and unresolved issues in regard to each life stage.[4] Matthew and Dennis Linn and Sheila Fabricant have built on Erikson's views to do retreats on the healing of memories. This work resulted in their book, *Healing the Eight Stages of Life.*[5] Their insights lead us to understand that midlife is not just an occasion for dealing with item 7 on Erikson's list; rather, it is the opportunity in adult years to reflect on all eight issues.

Erikson's theory has some problems, as we shall shortly note. Still, it is important both for what it says of enduring importance and for the further explorations it has triggered. Let us turn to another significant perspective.

DANIEL LEVINSON
The Seasons of a Man's Life

Daniel J. Levinson and his associates have investigated the stages of life from a different perspective. Erikson concentrated on unconscious processes in the development of adult identity. Levinson explored the conscious choices one makes regarding occupation, marriage, family, friends, and life goals.

Levinson and his colleagues did intensive interviews with forty men. Regretfully, they originally did not also interview women to compare their life stages (though their work has triggered parallel studies among women). The forty men were equally divided among four occupations: industrial laborers, biology professors, business executives, and novelists. Out of these interviews came a concept of life stages that is expressed in their work, *The Seasons of a Man's Life.*[6]

Levinson believes that the life cycle evolves through a series of eras, each of them approximately twenty-five years in duration. The sequence is as follows:

1. Childhood and adolescence: age 0–22
2. Early adulthood: age 17–45
3. Middle adulthood: age 40–65
4. Late adulthood: age 60–?[7]

According to Levinson, each era has its own distinctive and unifying qualities, like the act of a play or the major section of a novel. Of course, change and development do take place within each era.

One of Levinson's surprises was that development in adult years is age-linked.[8] While not everyone develops in exactly the same time sequence, he found that the age variations for the different eras did not vary by more than five or six years.

He concludes, then, that there is a *clearly identifiable, studyable progression of development for adults, just as there is for children and youth.*

On the border between each of the life stages, Levinson discovered that there is a "zone of overlap." That is the period when the old era is being completed and the new one is starting. This is not a simple, brief transition. Rather, it is a change of the fabric of one's life. Such transitions consistently take four or five years. The person's task in this time is to do the developmental work that links the eras and provides some continuity between them.

In broad outline, then, this is how Levinson diagrams the eras of a man's life:

Eras in the Male Life Cycle[9]

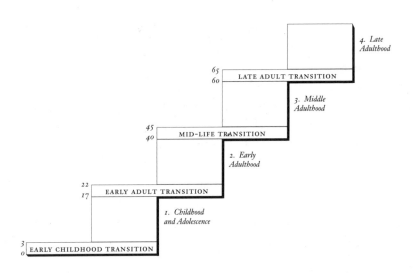

The basic developmental tasks of each of these periods of adult development (to age 50) are outlined below.[10]

EARLY ADULT TRANSITION: MOVING FROM
PRE-ADULTHOOD TO EARLY ADULTHOOD (AGES 17–22)

There are two tasks in this period. One is to start moving out of the pre-adult world, and the second is to make a preliminary step into the adult world. One must explore possibilities, imagine oneself as a participant in the adult world, and make preliminary choices for adult living.

THE FIRST ADULT STRUCTURE:
ENTERING THE ADULT WORLD (AGES 22–28)

A young adult has two basic, yet opposite, tasks: (a) to explore all the possibilities of adult living, and (b) to settle down and create a stable life structure—that is, to become responsible and "make something of oneself." These two tasks are so imperious, so contradictory, and so demanding that many young adults feel that they may have built a flawed life structure.

THE AGE THIRTY TRANSITION:
CHANGING THE FIRST LIFE STRUCTURE (AGES 28–33)

This five-year period provides an opportunity to work on the limitations and flaws of the first adult structure and to create something more satisfactory for the balance of early adulthood. For many in Levinson's study, there was an age thirty crisis—a time when one finds one's present life structure intolerable, yet finds oneself unable to formulate something better. When I told my story, I spoke of experiencing just such a crisis. This crisis is a time to ask, "What's missing that I want to add? What's inappropriate that I want to take out of my life?" In my opinion, midlife begins with these questions and with these possibly life-correcting decisions. These issues will return again and again.

THE SECOND ADULT LIFE STRUCTURE:
SETTLING DOWN (AGES 33–40)

Next, one may enter the settling-down period of a person's life calendar. There are two tasks in this period: (a) finding a niche in society and changing from a "novice" adult to one more firmly accepted, respected, and competent; and (b) "making it," that is, advancing in social rank, income, power, fame, creativity, quality of family life, social contribution, etc.

At the end of the Settling Down period, from about age thirty-six to forty, Levinson notes a distinctive phase he calls *Becoming*

One's Own Man (or, as he abbreviates it, BOOM!). The major developmental task here is to become a senior member in one's world—a person with a greater measure of authority.

THE MIDLIFE TRANSITION: MOVING FROM EARLY
TO MIDDLE ADULTHOOD (AGES 40–45)

In this transition period, the life structure again comes into question. One asks:

> What have I done with my life? What do I really get from and give
> to my [spouse], children, friends, work, community—and self?
> What is it I truly want for myself and others? What are my central
> values and how are they reflected in my life? What are my greatest
> talents and how am I using (or wasting) them? What have I done
> with my early Dream and what do I want with it now? Can I live in
> a way that combines my current desires, values and talents? How
> satisfactory is my present life structure—how suitable for the self,
> how viable in the world—and how shall I change it to provide a
> better basis for the future?[11]

For 80 percent of those interviewed, this transition was a time of moderate or severe crisis. It was so for me. I struggled with those questions Levinson noted—and many more. Nearly every aspect of one's life comes under scrutiny and questioning. A person will need several years to build a new life structure or modify an old one.

ENTERING MIDDLE ADULTHOOD:
BUILDING A NEW LIFE STRUCTURE (AGES 45–50)

One must now make one's choices and begin forming a new life structure. Levinson notes that those studied vary greatly in the success-appropriateness of the life structure they build at this time. Those who build an appropriate life pattern combine what is viable in the world and what is connected to the self they have discovered.[12]

He points out that there are *three aspects* of the developmental work of early and middle adulthood.[13] The *first* aspect is *building* and *modifying* the *life structure*. The second aspect is *working on single components* of the *life structure*. There are at least five such components:

1. *Forming and modifying a dream.* The early adult has formed a dream (relationally and occupationally). "In middle adulthood, one's task is to modify or give up the Dream."

2. *Forming and modifying an occupation.* Some people stay in a single occupation, but most make a few or many changes or have changes forced upon them.

3. *Love-marriage-family.* In many cases, interest in family increases with the middle years.

4. *Forming mentoring relationships.* As a young adult, one seeks a "mentor," one who is a teacher, a model, an influence on a person's life, an "admixture of good [parent] and good friend."[14] In midlife, one "fires" one's mentor and considers offering this same gift to yet others.

5. *Forming mutual friendships.* Levinson found that the men he studied had few male friends and even fewer nonsexual female friendships.

The third task is *adult individuation*, that is, the task of discovering "who I am in a unique sense." This involves dealing with at least four polarities, or opposite forces, in one's life:

1. *Young/old.* The middle adult needs to make sense of this in-between place in life.

2. *Destruction/creation.* The middle-aged person is more aware of coming death and of hurts that he or she has absorbed and inflicted. There is also a desire to become more creative and to contribute more fully to coming generations.

3. *Masculine/feminine.* In midlife, one needs to search for a more appropriate combination of "masculine" and "feminine" qualities in oneself.

4. *Attachment/separateness.* A major task of middle adulthood is to find a more appropriate balance between the needs of the self and the needs of society.

Just as this book was about to go to press, Daniel and Judy Levinson's new book, *The Seasons of a Woman's Life*, was released. (See Resources at end of chapter.) In it they apply their biographical interview methods to women, and they conclude that the basic theses—that human beings progress through life in predictable patterns and that development is a lifelong process—are again validated. The Levinsons do note some differences in women's life structure resulting from a rigid division between male and female, masculine and feminine, in human life. Some women accept this division, some pioneer in overcoming it, and some benefit because this phenomenon is changing and diminishing.

ROGER GOULD
Transformations

From quite different sources, Roger Gould developed an alternative view of life-stage tasks. He gained insights from supervising psychiatrists in training. Then he did subsequent research with persons who were not psychiatric patients. Out of this, Gould noted some age-related life issues that were different from those addressed in the two theories we have already cited. Gould noted:

> I concluded . . . that *adulthood is not a plateau*; rather, it is a dynamic and changing time for all of us. As we grow and change, we take steps *away* from childhood and *toward* adulthood—steps such as marriage, work, consciously developing a talent or buying a home. With each step, the unfinished business of childhood intrudes, disturbing our emotions and requiring psychological work. With this in mind, adults may now view their disturbed feelings at particular periods as a possible sign of progress, as part of their attempted movement toward a fuller adult life.[15]

Gould sees the adult as progressively correcting the misconceptions of what he calls *"childhood consciousness."* He points out that while most adults wistfully recall childhood as carefree and exuberant, they largely forget the other side of childhood. In childhood there is also "the powerful larger-than-life anger and hurt all children experience as they cope with the world."[16] Gould calls this potentially uncontrollable destructiveness "demonic anger." He suggests this demon, anger, is the key ingredient of childhood consciousness that must be mastered.

What triggers the demonic anger in adult life? Gould contends that both in children and in adults this anger is aroused each time we encounter a separation situation. For the child, it is a physical separation. For the adult, it is a love separation; that is, we feel misunderstood, mislabeled, or slighted.

"We are then faced with two realities: *current reality*—the reality of adult consciousness, the way we actually experience events and each other now; and *demonic reality*—the childhood consciousness reality, the intrusion into adult life of painful childhood states."[17]

This leads Gould to the basic thesis of his book: "*By striving for a fuller, more independent adult consciousness, we trigger the angry demons of childhood consciousness. Growing and reformulating our self-definition becomes a dangerous act. It is the act of transformation.*"[18]

In Gould's understanding, our adult consciousness evolves through a series of confrontations with our own childhood past. As adults, we become progressively more able to confront the demonic realities and to rework the irrationalities of childhood.

Gould suggests that the childhood consciousness is based on four major false assumptions that children make. They are the following:

1. We'll always live with our parents and be their child.
2. Our parents will always be there to help when we can't do something on our own.
3. Parents' simplified version of our complicated inner reality is correct, as when they turn the light on in our bedroom to prove there are no ghosts.
4. There is no real death or evil in the world.

Gould's understanding of adult life stages is that one of these assumptions is challenged in each stage of life.

The first assumption, "I'll always belong to my parents," comes under question during ages eighteen to twenty-two. At this time, the individual lives away from home and may take on beliefs or actions that don't fit the parental lifestyle and beliefs.

The second assumption, "They (my parents) will always be there to help me," is most powerfully challenged in our twenties.

A person begins to set up an independent life and make important decisions that no one else can make for an individual—career, marriage, pregnancy, etc. The person substitutes his or her own proven competence for the false assumption.

The third assumption, "Life is simple and controllable," is challenged in the late twenties and early thirties. At that time in life, "the simple rules and supposed-to-be's about life prove ineffectual in the complicated real world." When one challenges this assumption, one has moved into midlife, in my opinion.

The fourth assumption, "There is no evil or death in the world," is challenged in the late thirties through the fifties. Time pressures mount. Parents and other persons important to a person die. Children go out of one's life. The illusion (of no evil, death, or loss) must be destroyed if one is to face finitude and mortality with integrity and creativity. This issue is at the heart of many midlife struggles. This was an issue that haunted me around my fortieth birthday.

Gould's concept of life stages is that progressively through our lives, we come to grips with the "demons" of childhood consciousness. To the extent people succeed in shedding the assumptions of childhood, they are transformed into growing, becoming adults.

The Main Problem with These Theories

After surveying this literature, Carol Gilligan—former student and colleague of moral-development pioneer Lawrence Kohlberg —makes a crucial observation. She notes that nearly all of this discussion has been in the masculine domain. Men were either studied exclusively or given the major attention. "Then attempts have been made to interpret the lives of women through constructs derived from studies of men."[19]

She notes that Daniel Levinson begins by expressing distress that his study included only males. But he then proceeds to make a striking declaration. He sets out, he says, "to create an overarching conception of development that could encompass the diverse biological, psychological and social changes occurring in adult life."[20] He attempts to offer a comprehensive theory of life stages based on a study of representatives of one-half of the human race.

Further, Gilligan points out that Erikson's life tasks really don't fit the experience of women. He suggests that the central issue for youth is identity (who am I?); for the young adult it is intimacy (how and to whom can I relate?); for the middle adult it is generativity (how and whom can I mentor in a meaningful way?). That linear description does not fit women. For them, the issues of intimacy and identity are always closely intertwined. Indeed, identity is a social construct. We gain our identity from responses of others in community. Further, midlife is far too late for attention to generativity issues. One has probably had one's children and practically raised them by then!

She sees Levinson's and Erikson's theories as possible models for a healthy male life cycle for men who are achievers but are distant in their relationships. If they ever give attention to nurturing relationships, it is after their career goals have been reached. Such models will not fit all men; they will fit few or no women.

Further, Gilligan notes that as children and youths, males and females are socialized differently: "Female identity arises through attachment, through identification with the mother. . . . Male identity is contingent on separation from the mother and the reconstruction of the mother-son relationship in more differentiated . . . terms."[21] Therefore, male identity is defined through separation from women and connection to society (and thus to achievement). On the other hand, women's identity is defined personally in the ongoing continuity of relationships.

For both males and females entering young adult years, the issue is how to balance integrity of self and relationships with others. The male is socialized to emphasize one aspect, the female the other.

Therefore, developmental tasks—as well as the way they are approached—are apt to be different for females and males. Women's development may not be an orderly stair-step progression through life. It may more closely resemble "a braid of threads in which colors appear, disappear, and reappear."[22] Gilligan's perspective and critique, which she offered in 1982 in her ground-breaking book, *In a Different Voice: Psychological Theory and Women's Development,*[23] has stimulated considerable investigation and research into women's development—both by Gilligan herself and by colleagues.

Certainly, a healthy-life-cycle model derived from studies of only women would reveal something quite different from those for males that we cited above. For example, the psychiatrist Jean Baker Miller, in her studies of the psychology of women, noted women's sensitivity to others as well as their vulnerability to loss. Others had called these characteristics weaknesses, but Miller called them strengths.[24]

The theories of Erikson, Levinson, and Gould may offer women some insights and topics to consider. However, these perspectives cannot be definitive for women. This discovery leads to further questions. Has anyone successfully created a widely accepted life-stage theory for women? (not to my knowledge). If not, what might be the key elements of a view of life journeys for women? Several persons have made contributions in this regard. I will mention a few.

RUTHELLEN JOSSELSON
Finding Herself

Ruthellen Josselson reports on her longitudinal study (a study over a period of years with the same persons) in *Finding Herself.* In the early 1970s, she interviewed sixty randomly selected senior women from colleges and universities. Her focus was to understand how their adolescent identity formation influenced their lives. Twelve years later, she was able to locate and interview thirty-four of these women.

From the outset, it was clear to her that interpersonal competence was more important than autonomy to adolescent girls. Young women were less likely to separate forcefully from parents than young men. "In short, adolescent girls seem to formulate identity more in connection to others and at less distance from their families than do boys."[25]

In doing her original interviews, she found J. E. Marcia's four types of identity formation useful. These include:

1. *Identity foreclosure.* These young people make commitments in the absence of searching or crisis. They carry forward either parent expectations or childhood plans without subjecting them to question or scrutiny. This leads to a premature phase of development.
2. *Identity achievement.* These are young people who have tested options, lived with the questions, and then committed themselves to what they discovered.
3. *Moratorium.* These young people find themselves in a crisis or exploratory phase. They are struggling to find commitments that will engage them but have not found them yet.
4. *Identity diffusion.* These folks are drifting, perhaps avoiding the task of identity formation. They have abandoned childhood views but are not particularly looking for new ones.

As she reflected on her interviews twelve years later, Josselson wrote, "The configuration of a woman's identity at the close of adolescence forms the template for her adulthood."[26] Whatever identity-type category women were in at the end of formative college years tended to be where they still were.

Josselson notes that in the development of these women's self-identity, there is "the possibility that both achievement and interpersonal aspects of life are important."[27]

IRIS SANGIULIANO
In Her Time

Iris Sangiuliano is critical of life-stage theory because she believes it has limited usefulness for women. She criticizes the inadequacy of its predictability as not fitting women's experiences. Further, such theories do not allow for the unpredictable. She finds that critical events change the focus and direction of women's lives. She writes, "I was struck by the fact that women's lives unfold, not in a rigid, predictable, progression of conflicts, identity, mastery, and autonomy, but rather in great surges of billowing changes."[28]

Sangiuliano interviewed a number of middle-class midlife women who were presently married or who had been. (Her interviews took place in the mid 1970s.) For women of that generation, she noted a slower, more arduous development for women than for men. She contended that men were groomed to *do*, while women were taught to *be*. The women she interviewed were "late bloomers" who postponed themselves. They expected to be married, and they succeeded in accomplishing that. They first thought in terms of "we." And then, at some time, they discovered the "I" within the "we" (or outside it).

How does this emergence of the "I" occur? Sangiuliano quotes sculptor Louise Nevelson: "Most of us have to be transplanted, like a tree, before we blossom."[29] Disruption, contradiction, paradox—these can be the occasions for growth and self-discovery.

Sangiuliano approvingly cites the theory of Klaus Riegel. Riegel pointed out that adult development includes movement along four dimensions. An unexpected crisis in any of these four dimensions may stir major upheavals, disruptions, and transformations in a woman's life. The four dimensions are:

1. *Inner-biological.* For example, the discovery of a life-threatening illness.
2. *Individual-psychological.* For example, a woman may discover that she cannot bury herself in her husband's or anybody else's identity.
3. *Cultural-sociological.* This is the discovery that one is out of step with one's social environs. For example, a woman whose husband had joined the back-to-earth movement and had bought a farm discovers she has no interest in baking bread or making sausage.
4. *Outer-physical.* For example, wars, floods, famines, pestilences.

"In short, unless we disrupt the old and the familiar and suffer the disenchantments, there's no room for the new."[30]

JOANNE F. VICKERS AND BARBARA L. THOMAS
No More Frogs, No More Princes

Joanne Vickers and Barbara Thomas interviewed over one hundred women between the ages of forty and sixty about their experiences with a midlife transition. Their research was conducted fifteen to twenty years after Sangiuliano's and with persons in a wider range of ethnic and economic circumstances, yet their findings are remarkably similar. Out of their research, they reported that twenty of the persons they interviewed had found ways to make creative choices for the rest of their lives.

They found that the creativity chosen by these women fell into three categories. The first group chose a traditional outlet in the arts—for example, painting or pottery—to express themselves. Creativity through art also helped the individual get in touch with her identity, which was a source of great joy.

The second group—the majority—became involved in new work and/or new affiliations. This might be marriage, volunteer work, or a new career. These persons found a new sense of personal power and fulfillment in these relationships or tasks.

The third group focused on developing their inner lives. Their focus was to create a life that is inner-directed, that is, spiritual. They rearranged lifestyles; they allowed time for silence and reflection. For them, creativity is as much letting go as it is taking on new ventures.

How does one go about making creative choices? Vickers and Thomas interpreted the experiences of the people they interviewed through a paradigm from *The Creative Spirit* by Daniel Goleman, Paul Kaufman, and Michael Ray.[31] This paradigm consists of four stages.

- It begins with *preparation*. For a woman, this preparation may begin with the awareness that the relationships in which she has invested herself all her life are coming to be less fulfilling. Something else is needed to make life rich and meaningful. An awareness of physical limitations may dawn upon her as well, bringing a sense of urgency.
- Next there is *incubation*. Information and experiences sink into the unconscious, where they grow into new ideas and images. This process just happens. There is nothing that can be done to make it work. Waiting is essential to well-being.

- Incubation is followed by *illumination*. This may seem to be very sudden—an "aha!" moment, a bolt out of the blue. Actually it emerges from the two previous processes. This moment of illumination can both delight and frighten a person. It can heighten one's dissatisfaction with life as it is, but it can force one's attention on the need for changes in one's life, perhaps drastic changes. Psychologist Marsha Sinetar notes, "Letting go of all that is dear or familiar can be our starting point of power. When we leap into an abyss in order to honor life . . . we experience rebirth as a larger, mysteriously expanded self."[32]

- Finally, there is *translation*. Out of this self-discovery and realization, the person takes risks to translate dreams into reality.

As with any creative process, as we women give shape to our midlife identity, we realize a sure joy, a grace, and a sense of rightness with ourselves and the world. It is in midlife that women can come to understand and shape their own stories.[33]

MAGGIE SCARF
Unfinished Business

Each of the feminist writers above spoke of the importance of intimacy and relationships in a woman's identity formation through time. Scientific writer and journalist Maggie Scarf makes a similar discovery. In attempting to understand depression in women, she had a fascinating conversation with Marcia Guttentag, a psychologist. Guttentag had been conducting a content analysis of major themes in men's and in women's popular magazines. She noted that the stories for men were primarily concerned with adventures, achievement, and triumph over difficult odds. By contrast, the central theme of stories in the women's magazines was coping with loss. Scarf built on this discovery to write her book, *Unfinished Business*. She describes women's development through an understanding of the centrality of relationships. Scarf also explores the critical losses that occur at each stage. In summary, Scarf writes:

The replies I was getting varied—in relatively systematic ways—with the various stages of the life cycle. . . . Women in the same phase of life were, by and large, depressed about similar sorts of things.

In adolescence . . . with such matters as the wrench of separation from one's parents, and with changing body image—the frightening journey of transformation from child to sexual woman.

In the years of the twenties . . . with the search for intimacy and commitment: the career costs that might be incurred, should one put the "loving" tasks ahead of the work ones—or indeed, should one do things the opposite way around!

Issues of the thirties were, frequently, the mistakes that had already been made and the payment that had been exacted: an "I've been cheated" sense that the fantasies and dreams of girlhood had not been and might never *be* satisfied.

At mid-life, major preoccupations were with the loss of certain identity-conferring roles or ways of being—roles which, in many an instance, had been perceived as a person's sole source of interpersonal power or meaning. It might be the fading of a woman's attractiveness. . . . Or it might be that a woman's depressive symptoms had emerged around the departure of a child, perhaps the youngest child—and the subsequent loss of the nurturing mothering role which she'd conceived of as her identity, her reason for being.[34]

Scarf offers a view of a woman's life journey as a search for intimacy and the effort to cope with the losses that inevitably occur. Each of these authors offers key issues and themes of which one must be aware in attempting to understand women's journeys through life. From a dialogue among these persons, an alternative view of women's life journey and life stages begins to emerge.

These observations strike an important note: An understanding of human growth and maturity should be built on women's studies, men's studies, and dialogues between them.

SOMETHING MORE—
BABY BOOMERS ARE NOW IN MIDLIFE!

Social scientists use the term "cohorts" to describe groups of people whose birth dates have something in common. This may be within a given decade or within a given era. I was born in the "cohort" of depression babies. Birth rates were very low. Early memories included real drought and unemployment and even more stories about it. I remember WPA workers constructing a road with hand shovels in front of the house where we lived. World events that impacted childhood and youth in my cohort were World War II, the death of President Roosevelt, the atomic bomb. Because my cohort was a relatively small group, we were not particularly noted or provided for by society. When I came to the pain of midlife issues, research on such matters was sparse. My cohort was not large enough to demand attention, so I found very few helpful resources.

By contrast, those born between 1946 and 1964 are the cohort of "baby boomers." A broad-based postwar economic prosperity lasting more than twenty years fueled this boom. Americans married at early ages and raised larger families, which were affordable in the affluence of those years. Fully one-third of the American population, approximately 75 million persons, are part of this cohort. Because of its size, this cohort has needed a variety of expanded services—schools, for example. And commercial enterprises have catered to this group's needs.[35]

This cohort is better informed about emerging life-development theory than were previous generations. As he observes the intersection of baby boomers and midlife, John Roschen observes, "[M]idlife is bound to be fascinating territory for they will make of it something more—expansive, they will extend it—as they have of everything they have ever done throughout their lifetimes."[36]

The baby boomer generation also has reason to be skeptical about some aspects of life-stage theory and to reframe it in light of their own experience. Those studies by men and women from the

1970s do not entirely coincide with the boomers' experience. Speaking as a baby boomer, psychologist Ross Goldstein writes,

> This core principle of stage theory is crumbling under the weight of numerous social trends initiated by the baby boom generation. Life schedules today resemble anything but a straight-line march. For our generation, the identity crisis that Erikson thought should be resolved in adolescence now often persists well into the twenties; the bonding stage that is thought to typically occur in the mid-twenties may be delayed until the thirties, or experienced more than once. People who have pursued careers with a vengeance may find the generativity crisis coming earlier than it's supposed to; and people of advanced age may be too busy with a second marriage or a third career to evaluate ego integrity.
>
> The changes in women's life patterns, in particular, demonstrate the increasing irrelevance of stage theory centered on age. Women entering the work place en masse, delaying marriage and child birth, and the many women beginning careers in midlife have thrown these predictable tasks and crises way off schedule. "Give me a roomful of 40-year-old women," declares adult development observer Nancy Schlossberg, "and you have told me nothing."[37]

Cheryl Merser heartily concurs. When she read Gail Sheehy's *Passages*—a popular summary of Erikson-Levinson-Gould, and more—she was puzzled. It described her parents' generation very well. However, it was not at all accurate in speaking of her and her generation. Poignantly she asks,

> How . . . can you have a career crisis if you haven't found the right career or even a job? How can you feel trapped by a mortgage if you can't afford a house? How can you have a seven-year marital itch if you're still single by the time you're thirty? How can you have an all-out mid-life crisis at thirty-five if you're attending your first Lamaze class? How can you suffer the empty-nest syndrome if you're childless and approaching forty? How can you deal with the predictable ups and downs of a marriage if both of

you are working all the time and never see each other? And most important, if we can't use the benchmarks of another generation to guide us through the life cycle, what benchmarks are we to use instead?[38]

Merser aptly entitles her book *"Grown Ups": A Generation in Search of Adulthood.* She points out another area in which earlier theories do not apply. Midlife has been seen as the time when males get in touch with their gentler, nurturing, "female" side, and as a time when women get in touch with their assertive, aggressive, "male" side. She suggests that there is a new life-cycle "formula" for men and women in the first half of life today. Both men and women are taught to care about others, and also to be competitive. And so upon reaching maturity, men and women no longer "complement" each other. Rather, they compete with each other. The competition exists in the marketplace for jobs and status, and also in the home for the emotional space and support that each person needs.[39] This implies a new way of working out one's life agenda and needs—whether one is male or female. It also points to a new kind of marriage—two equals working hard to provide for both their own and the other's needs.

Gail Sheehy has recently returned to the subject of life stages nearly twenty years after she published *Passages.* Her new book is entitled *New Passages: Mapping Your Life Across Time.*[40] In it, Sheehy totally agrees with the critiques such as those Goldstein and Merser bring—that it does not fit their generation. Her vast research unearths even greater changes. She points out that age norms have shifted and are no longer normative. People are leaving childhood sooner, staying in adolescence longer, and delaying midlife by a substantial period of time. While it might be roughly accurate to add ten years to every life stage she suggested in her earlier volume, she suggests that life's passages are far more complex than that.

She points out that for centuries the human life cycle has been defined by bearing and caring for children. With modern technology people are deferring childbirth for ten to twenty years. This, she says, renders any expectation of a uniform life course incoherent.

And so there is no longer a standard life cycle. People are increasingly able to customize their life cycles. All of this change has its cost—namely, we are cut off from the wisdom of the ages and of preceding generations as to how to age. This may lead to a suspension from our spiritual selves. We may understand our lives less and less.[41]

With all these disclaimers, Sheehy still feels that a major life passage occurs somewhere around one's mid-forties. She sees this as transition into what she calls "second adulthood." She feels that the second adulthood has two distinct periods. The first is the years from approximately 45 to 65, which she terms the "age of mastery." The second is the years of late adulthood from 65 to 85 or beyond, which she terms the "age of integrity."

The basic task for entering this second adulthood is to construct a new second adult identity. This may involve casting off an identity that was based on the assumptions and expectations of others and developing clarity about that which is life-giving and life-renewing for the rest of one's lifetime.[42]

While most life-stage theories emphasize the individual, we do not age in a vacuum. A number of factors, many of them beyond our control, will enter into our life experience. These factors will influence our degree of success in fulfilling our lifetime aspirations—and, to an extent, what those aspirations are. Some of these are: economic booms, busts, or recessions; wars, including possible military conscription; trends such as urbanization; the decline of an occupation for which one has interest or preparation, or the rapid rise in the need for one's occupation; the rise of technologies (for example, the computer) with which one must come to grips; movements, such as civil rights, feminism, or the peace movement; and the relative size of one's age cohort.

It is true that one must negotiate the changes of which life stage theories speak. However, one will do so in the midst of a number of outside circumstances. These matters may delay, interfere with, or dramatically alter those tasks. For the baby boom generation, there are a few additional twists.

FURTHER, WE LIVE LONGER

We need to revise our thinking in the light of increased life expectancy. In 1900, the average American could expect to live forty-seven years. The average length of a person's life in the United States has increased by almost 60 percent during this century. By 1992, a male's life expectancy had climbed to seventy-three years and a female's to eighty.[43] The average life expectancy for women may well increase to 90 or more. Half of all Americans who have ever lived past the age of sixty-five are alive now. The fastest-growing age segment in this country is those over eighty-five.

We live in a period marked by the discovery of healthful diets, aerobic exercise, the reduction of tobacco use, and increased medical resources for all ages. (Health issues will be explored in the next chapter.) Thus it is reasonable to envision that life expectancy will increase even more.

This expectation impacts the experience of midlife more than one might first think. For openers, it alters the time at which midlife begins. Bernice Neugarten once suggested that midlife had arrived when one quit measuring time from one's birth and started measuring time until one's death. If reasonable life expectancies grow ten years in one's lifetime, does midlife delay five years? One would think so. Indeed, in a recent survey, persons were asked when midlife begins. The average answer was age forty-six.[44] Or perhaps midlife extends both ways—to the entire middle third of life, ages thirty to sixty or thereabouts.

Not only is life expanding, but with health and cosmetic options for both women and men, youthfulness is also extending. In some ways actual youthful vigor is lasting longer.

Karen Blaker explores this topic in her book, *Celebrating Fifty*. She speaks of discovering—first in herself, then in others whom she interviewed—how the experience of being a woman in one's fifties has changed.

I realized that a shift of monumental proportions had taken place in the way women relate to reaching the turning point of fifty. Most of the women who have shared their experiences with me have said that they don't feel in the least bit over-the-hill. Their time lines for aging have changed, even if society at large has not yet adjusted to the change. With life expectancies for healthy American women now averaging more than eighty years, women of fifty refuse to be called old.[45]

Blaker discovered a parallel issue that went with experiencing youthful vigor in one's fifties. There was the lack of guidance for living one's life appropriately. She points to the "humor" contained in birthday cards about being fifty: (a) On the cover of a card, "There's something to be said about turning fifty"; inside the card, "It sucks." (b) "Don't worry about this birthday . . . fifty isn't old . . . If you're a tree." (c) "How many fifty-year-olds does it take to change a light bulb? None. They prefer it dark. Better for napping."[46]

However, beyond these conceptions of aging as an illness is the fact there are few role models to follow. Those in generations before us did—for the most part—feel, look, and act older than many of us at the same age. How are we to conduct ourselves with appropriate vigor and dignity?

Not only are there few role models, there is such a thin line between healthy and unhealthy behaviors and attitudes. We live in a youth-affirming, sometimes youth-worshiping, society. An important concern of midlife is the recognition that one *is* losing some of one's youthfulness and becoming older. The bizarre behavior sets in when one attempts to repress that aging process. That is when those afflicted with the "midlife crazies" cannot face the fact that they are aging. When one ignores or denies one's age, inappropriate dress, behavior, acting out may well occur.

It is healthy to affirm life, to enhance life, to extend life, to enjoy youthfulness into one's mature years. But it is unhealthy to repress that one is aging. It is unhealthy to worship at the altar of youthfulness so that one does not celebrate one's later life stages.

However, one must do sensitive reflection to separate one behavior from the other.

There is yet another aspect of midlife issues that has changed with increased life expectancy. The anticipated life spans of one's parents has also increased. This means that care for the generation before us may well continue throughout all of our midyears and into our retirement. Indeed, about 10 percent of those over age sixty-five also have children who are over sixty-five![47] Quite likely, this percentage will grow. (I will speak in much more detail about this in chapter 7.)

The fact of growing life expectancy impacts the experience of midlife in myriad ways.

MORE VARIATIONS

We need to realize that midlife adjustments have more variations than some theories imply. There are at least two major ways of looking at the adult life span. One way is to emphasize stages and transitions as Erikson, Levinson, and Gould do. Another way is to focus on the timing of the events that one faces. This approach does not look for (or find) such clearly marked developmental steps.

Janet Zollinger Giele recognizes these widely divergent ways of describing adult aging. She then asks whether one of these perspectives is truer than the other. Giele answers that probably each theory is correct but limited in its explanatory power. She suggests that each theory, perhaps, applies to different types of people and circumstances.

She notes that most stage theorists are psychologists or psychoanalysts who work with an educated, sophisticated, privileged segment of society. On the other hand, nonstage theorists tend to be trained in sociology and look at a broader spectrum of society. Giele concludes:

> Evidently some people experience distinct stages of adult development while others do not. It is the degree of social complexity on the job or in other aspects of everyday life that appears critical.

Those who must learn a great deal and adapt to many different roles seem to be the most concerned with trying to evolve an abstract self, conscience, or life structure that can integrate all these discrete events. By contrast, those with a simple job, limited by meager education and narrow contacts, are less apt to experience aging as a process that enhances autonomy or elaborates one's mental powers.[48]

In addition to Giele's contribution, there are other reasons for different interpretations of the aging process. Different personality types are apt to encounter midlife differently. For example, the Myers-Briggs personality test, which is built on Jung's personality theory, offers four contrasts. One of these is that a person is either Intuitive (N) or Sensing (S) in taking in information. The Intuitive person looks within the self. The Sensing person looks outside to what can be seen, touched, tasted, felt, or heard. There are two ways to process information, Thinking or Feeling. Thinking persons use objective logic without reference to how decisions affect others. Feeling persons consider their own and others' feelings in deciding how to act.

A Sensing-Thinking (ST) midlife person may be aware there are some *exterior* changes in his or her living circumstance that need to be managed. An Intuitive-Feeling (NF) midlife person will instead listen to what is going on *inside* the self as aging, losses, and decisions confront him or her.

Each of these two personality types is likely to misunderstand the other at this stage of life. The Intuitive-Feeling person may suspect that the Sensing-Thinking person is denying or repressing the pain of inner midlife issues. The Sensing-Thinking person may wonder why the Intuitive-Feeler is making such a fuss about such a simple thing as a fortieth birthday! This in part accounts for the very different attitudes toward fortieth birthdays of my spouse, Mary Ann, and me, that I mentioned in the previous chapter. Mary Ann is an ST, according to Myers-Briggs; I am an NF.

In progressing through midlife, there are at least two distinct areas of concern. There is the area of outer responsibility. This includes marriage, possibly divorce or widowhood (including providing for one's needs as a single), and parenting. It involves helping young adult children become launched and coping when they return home. It also includes career moves and direction, retirement planning, working out one's changing financial needs, dealing with one's aging parents, and more.

Then there is the area of inner responsibility. This includes accepting oneself as an older adult, coping with loss and change, coming to grips with one's finitude and death. It further entails wrestling with a faith adequate for these crises, evolving a maturing spirituality, and more.

Each of us needs to be in touch with both the inner and the outer issues of midlife. It is a mistake to let one aspect drown out the other. Only by living with all dimensions of midlife will one experience all the potential growth this stage of life offers. In this book we will look first at the outer issues and then at the inner issues.

William Bridges raises yet another issue about the theories we have been exploring. He was attracted to them at first, but he has become more skeptical. "My work with individuals in transition," he writes, "makes me believe that in a culture as diverse as ours, no one model of adulthood fits everyone—or even anyone—exactly."[49] Rather, he sees all of adulthood as "a rhythm of expansion and contraction, change and stability." In this process, the constant feature is a series of endings, followed by a "neutral zone" and then a beginning.[50] He feels that rather than having one big midlife crisis, which so many assume, adults may more aptly be seen as going through a series of transitions, which an individual negotiates wisely or foolishly.

THE SPIRITUAL-RELIGIOUS-THEOLOGICAL
DIMENSION OF MIDLIFE

We need to give the spiritual-religious-theological dimension of midlife the central focus it deserves. When speaking to a group of psychiatrists about his life-stage research, Daniel Levinson was asked an interesting question. Did his researchers explore the religious dimension of the men they interviewed in depth? He responded that they raised no questions about religious life, but if a subject chose to talk about religion, he was allowed to do so. Clearly, religious development was not given a central spot in Levinson's research. Nor was it, as far as one can discern, in the other midlife theories we have described. And yet each of them is marked by an implicit religious dimension.

When Levinson wrote *The Seasons of a Man's Life*, he spoke of finitude, of the stewardship of time, and of a pilgrimage through life. His title calls to mind the psalmist's prayer: "So teach us to count our days that we may gain a wise heart" (Ps. 90:12).

There are possible theological concerns in Erikson's categories. He speaks of the adult issues of identity (image of God); intimacy (koinonia-fellowship and love); generativity (renewal, revival, discipling, and new birth); and integrity (dominion of God and hope).

When Gould speaks of "transformations," which come when we overcome the "demons" of childhood consciousness, he is speaking in theological terms. Quite likely Gould is consciously giving psychological interpretation to these belief terms. But we who read Gould's works with eyes of faith can turn the tables as well. We live in fellowship with the one who casts out demons. Indeed, he once cast out a demon in answer to a desperate cry, "I believe; help my unbelief!" (Mark 9:24).

There are those who see religious concerns at the very heart of the midlife experience. Karl Jung, truly the grandfather of all theorists of midlife, once wrote:

> Among all my patients in the second half of life—that is to say, over thirty five—there has not been one whose problem in the last resort was not that of finding a religious outlook on life.[51]

Further, he called on churches to provide guidance.

> I have just said that we have no schools for forty-year-olds. That is not quite true. Our religions were always such schools in the past, but how many people regard them as such today? How many of us

older persons have really been brought up in such a school and prepared for the second half of life, for old age, death and eternity?[52]

Jung spoke prophetically at this point. A religious perspective has much to offer and much to learn from dialogue with people in midlife transition. In this volume, I will offer theological reflection from time to time. I will also speak of spiritual growth in chapter 9 and offer a theology of midlife in chapter 10. A religious perspective should stand at the heart of a study of life stages if the exploration is to be complete.

With awareness of the richness, variety, and diversity of people experiencing midlife, we now examine the most frequent issues we midlifers encounter.

For Personal or Group Reflection and Discussion

1. On a piece of paper, draw a "time line" of your life to date.
   - Put your birth date on one end, the present date on the other.
   - Note important events along the time line, such as births, graduations, geographical moves, job changes, marriages, divorces, deaths, etc.
   - List events that may be more inward, but important to you. This might include steps of faith, key discoveries or ideas, experiences of counseling or therapy, etc.
   - Draw a line connecting these events—draw the line any way you want to.
   - If it seems fitting, divide your life into "eras," like the chapters in a book. Give each "chapter" a name.

2. If you are willing, compare your time line with those of other persons of your same sex and then with those of persons of the opposite sex.

3. Compare the events on your time line with what the various authors cited in this chapter say about life journeys and life tasks. Does one of their descriptions come closer to your experience than the others?

4. Are you a baby boomer? If so, how does this impact your experience of midlife?

5. What part does faith play in dealing with your life journey?

Resources

American Board of Family Practice. *Perspectives on Middle Age: The Vintage Years.* Lexington, Ky.: American Board of Family Practice, 1990.

Blaker, Karen. *Celebrating Fifty.* Chicago: Contemporary Books, 1990.

Brennan, Anne, and Janice Brewi. *Mid-Life Directions.* New York: Paulist Press, 1985.

Brewi, Janice, and Anne Brennan. *Midlife.* New York: Paulist Press, 1982.

Bridges, William. *Transitions.* Reading, Mass.: Addison-Wesley, 1980.

Erikson, Erik. *Childhood and Society.* New York: W. W. Norton and Co., 1950.

Ford, Iris M. *Life Spirals: The Faith Journey.* Burlington, Ont.: Welch Publishing Company, 1988, 1990.

Giele, Janet Zollinger. "Women in Adulthood: Unanswered Questions." In *Women in the Middle Years*, ed. Janet Zollinger Giele, 1–36. New York: John Wiley and Sons, 1982.

Gilligan, Carol. "Adult Development and Women's Development: Arrangements for a Marriage." In *Women in the Middle Years*, ed. Janet Zollinger Giele, 89–114. New York: John Wiley and Sons, 1982.

———. *In a Different Voice: Psychological Theory and Women's Development.* Cambridge: Harvard University Press, 1982(b).

Goldstein, Ross, with Diana Landau. *Fortysomething.* Los Angeles: Jeremy P. Tarcher, 1990.

Goleman, Daniel, Paul Kaufman, and Michael Ray. *The Creative Spirit.* New York: Dutton Publishers, 1992.

Gould, Roger L. *Transformations.* New York: Simon and Schuster, 1978.

Hawley, Gwen. *Measures of Psychosocial Development.* Odessa, Tex.: Psychological Assessment Resources, Inc., 1988.

Josselson, Ruthellen. *Finding Herself: Pathways to Identity Development in Women.* San Francisco: Jossey-Bass, 1987.

Levinson, Daniel, Charlotte N. Darrow, Edward B. Klein, Maria H. Levinson, and Braxton McKee. *The Seasons of a Man's Life.* New York: Alfred A. Knopf, 1978.

Levinson, Daniel J., in collaboration with Judy D. Levinson. *The Seasons of a Woman's Life.* New York: Alfred A. Knopf, 1996.

Life Insurance Fact Book. Washington, D.C.: American Council of Life Insurance, 1994.

Linn, Matthew, Dennis Linn, and Sheila Fabricant. *Healing the Eight Stages of Life*. New York: Paulist Press, 1988.

McCoy, Vivian Rogers, Colleen Ryan, and James W. Lichtenberg. *The Adult Life Cycle*. Lawrence, Kans.: Adult Life Center, Division of Continuing Education, 1978, 1979.

Merser, Cheryl. *"Grown Ups": A Generation in Search of Adulthood*. New York: G. P. Putnam's Sons, 1987.

Neugarten, Bernice, ed. *Middle Age and Aging*. Chicago: University of Chicago Press, 1968.

Olson, Richard P. *Mid-Life: A Time to Discover, A Time to Decide*. Valley Forge, Pa.: Judson Press, 1980.

Roschen, John Franklin. *Baby Boomers Face Midlife: Implications for Faith Communities in the Nineties and Beyond*. Prepared for Adult Faith Resources, Minneapolis, 1991.

Rountree, Cathleen. *Coming into Our Fullness: On Women Turning Forty*. Freedom, Calif.: The Crossing Press, 1991.

Sangiuliano, Iris. *In Her Time*. New York: William Morrow, 1978.

Scarf, Maggie. *Unfinished Business: Pressure Points in the Lives of Women*. New York: Doubleday, 1980.

Seasons of Life. Videotape. The Annenberg CPB Collection. Santa Barbara, Calif.: Intellimatch, 1990.

Sheehy, Gail. *Passages*. New York: E. P. Dutton, 1974.

———. *New Passages*. New York: Random House, 1995.

Treas, Judith, and Vern L. Bengston. "The Demography of Mid- and Late-Life Transitions." In Felix M. Berardo, ed., *Middle and Late Life Transitions: The Annals of the American Academy of Political and Social Science*, vol. 464 (Nov. 1982): 11–21. Beverly Hills: Sage Publications.

Troll, Lillian E. "Family Life in Middle and Old Age: The Generation Gap." In Felix M. Berardo, ed., *Middle and Late Life Transitions: The Annals of the American Academy of Political and Social Science*, vol. 464 (Nov. 1982): 38–46. Beverly Hills: Sage Publications.

Vickers, Joanne F., and Barbara L. Thomas. *No More Frogs, No More Princes: Women Making Creative Choices at Midlife*. Freedom, Calif.: The Crossing Press, 1993.

Whitehead, Evelyn Eaton, and James D. Whitehead. *Christian Life Patterns*. Garden City, N.Y.: Doubleday and Company, Inc., 1979.

II

Outer Journeys
in the
Middle Years

2

Health
Management

S O FAR, WE HAVE LOOKED at the adult life cycle, both individually and in overview considera- tion. I now invite your attention to a series of issues that we will face throughout our adult years. The first of these is health.

We who have lived through the 1960s, 1970s, 1980s, and into the 1990s have witnessed a revolution in health awareness.

In the early '60s, President John F. Kennedy personified phys- ical activity and fitness. Images of him playing touch football, running along beaches, or taking fifty-mile hikes influenced American consciousness and behavior. Indeed, he was said to be surprised that this modeling of behavior was more influential than his leadership on some national policies.

In 1968, a former Air Force doctor, Kenneth Cooper, wrote a landmark book, *Aerobics*. It gave people numbers to work with for exercise, fitness, and health. Dr. Cooper offered guidance as to how much exercise was beneficial and offered easy-to-follow ac- tivities. Many were surprised at how little exercise was needed to bring about substantial health benefits.

In 1972, persons watching network television coverage of the Olympic Games in Munich, Germany, found a new hero. A skinny young man—128 pounds, a Yale Law School student—did something no American had done for fifty years: Frank Shorter won the grueling twenty-six-mile marathon. This stimulated the running revolution, which expanded with extensive coverage of the 1976 Montreal Olympics.

Through the 1980s and now in the '90s, all sorts of methods to enhance healthy living are both available and popular. Richard Benyo and Rhonda Provost describe the present scene:

> Aerobic dance, strength training, triathlons, body-building, home gyms, leg warmers, twenty-four-hour clubs. The running revolution of the late 1970s, thought to be a fad that would pass, has evolved into an American mania that the rest of the world is emulating. Fitness, health, feeling better, looking better, using sports and physical exercise as an outlet in an office-oriented world, making positive efforts to delay the onslaught of aging—fitness integrated with daily life has become a new and refreshing lifestyle.[1]

That's the good news. Important information about improving adult health is now available. It is contributing to longevity, offering zest and more enjoyment of living. This health wisdom has now been widely available for more than twenty years. Ways of using it have been widely marketed and consumed by many.

However, we must add that it has been a rather uneven revolution. As with so many things that are good for us, many of us *know* far more than we *do*. Further, with so many sporting events on television, we may sometimes delude ourselves. We sports lovers may think that we are active because we are interested in sports, and watch sports for many hours!

Each middle adult will need to assess his or her own health habits. Then, each of us will need to decide what changes, if any, to make. As I have been sorting this out for myself, there are several considerations that come to mind.

For one thing, *I alone am responsible for the health management habits that will impact my health.* Only I can choose, and only I can follow through on those decisions. There is much about my health that I cannot control. I did not pick my gender or my genes.

Either because of my genetic inheritance or for yet other reasons, there may be potential or present health hazards in my body. I can't control that. Nor can I control some aspects of my environment (which may be healthy or not). Still, every reasonable decision that I *can* make about my health is mine alone to make.

Then again, *to make effective health decisions and to follow through is hard work. It is also a long-term, lifetime commitment.* It is important that we realize this. In this day of instant everything, there are those who falsely promise instant health solutions. Some weight-loss programs promise this. They suggest that in a matter of weeks, they will help me solve a weight problem that was twenty years in the making! Healthy living is hard work. It requires discipline. It should be undertaken as a lifelong commitment. To be sure, there will be steps of growth and steps backward. There are no quick fixes or instant solutions to health issues.

Further, *even the best health plan will not prevent my aging process.* Good health habits can slow down a rapid aging process that poor practices are accelerating. Good practices can lengthen that road to bodily aging. However, nothing can prevent it. I recall a delightful ninety-five-year-old man, Oliver, telling the doctor at his bedside, "I have something you can't cure—old age." Indeed, the doctor could not, for old age is not a disease. It is a condition. Aging is a process that begins at my birth and continues all my days. Oliver postponed it about as well as any person I ever knew. At age ninety-four, he crafted beautiful clock cabinets and cooked his own meals. He loved preparing special dishes for church potluck suppers. He enjoyed relating and joking with persons of all ages. But Oliver did not escape the aging process. No one does.

To continue, *the best of health habits will not prevent my eventual death. Life is a terminal condition. I will die someday.* Ironically, my awareness of my eventual demise may be one of the healthiest stimulants available to me. Once I recognize this body as a temporary apparatus, I will care for it more and abuse it less. If I have avoided or ignored this topic, I may continue many unhealthy practices that will drag my body down. I may continue to rationalize: "There's nothing you can do—when your time is up, it's up."

Rather, aware of my mortality, I will do well to envision a stamp on my physical health: "Fragile—Handle with Care."

After the previous somber comments, I add one on a more positive note. *I choose good health habits not only to increase the quantity of my life but to enhance the quality of my life.* I agree with the statement, "The purpose of fitness is to add more life to years, not just years to life." I want a lifestyle in which I feel good, look good, in which I am vibrant, sexy, fully alive.

With these basic considerations, let us proceed. We will look first at two major families of diseases with which we contend in our middle and later years. Next we will look specifically at health practices that are indicated in the light of these threats. Then we will conclude by returning to a broad perspective on personal health.

Health and One's Cardiovascular System

The cardiovascular system includes the heart and all the blood vessels in our body. It is an amazing pump and delivery system. This system brings nutrients to and takes waste from every single part of the body.

When this system functions well, we have the energy and alertness to do all the things important to us. It is a wonderful system, an unseen blessing. It is also crucially important to our actions, our thinking—indeed, our life itself.

A disease of this system, atherosclerosis, is a major cause of all deaths. This disease occurs when the inner layers of an artery are made much smaller. In turn oxygen-rich blood is not carried to that part of the body where the blockage occurs. Then that organ (or part of it) dies. Thus, if coronary arteries are blocked, the heart is not supplied with enough blood to sustain life. As a result, part or all of the heart muscle dies. If blockage occurs in the blood vessels to the brain, death occurs to that section of the brain deprived of oxygen.

As a result of atherosclerosis, heart attack and stroke are the biggest causes of death in the United States. About 47 percent of all deaths come from these illnesses. The sheer numbers are startling. Americans still feel the anguish of the Vietnam War, in which 57,000 Americans were killed; by contrast, heart disease kills *550,000 people*, every year, many of them in their most productive years.

Medical practitioners have noted that careful prevention of atherosclerosis can add perhaps twenty years to one's life, possibly even more. This precaution can contribute even more to the quality of those years.

You would think that with such a massive killing disease, there would be an urgent search to find the causes. Further, one would expect that, once found, these causes would be urgently stamped out. The tragic truth is that the causes are largely known, but all too often they are ignored until the damage is done.

Every single handbook on cardiovascular health lists virtually the same nine—or so—causes. A few of them are beyond the individual's control. Most of them are well within one's choice and decision. Here is that list of causes:

1. *High levels of serum cholesterol* was long suspected as a factor in the closing of blood vessels. In 1984, extensive federally sponsored studies indicated that lowering serum-cholesterol levels can substantially reduce the risk of heart disease. This can be done through diet, and, if needed, by medication.

2. *Hypertension* (high blood pressure—diastolic reading over 90) is clearly a major contributor to heart disease. This, too, can be altered by lifestyle decisions about weight, diet, and exercise, and by medication.

3. *Cigarette smoking* dramatically increases the risk of heart disease.

These three, all preventable and/or treatable (at least in part) are the biggest causes. In combination, the danger increases. One study revealed that people aged 30 to 59 with none of these health hazards had very little danger of a stroke. If a person had one of the hazards, there were 48 chances in 1000 of stroke; two of them, ninety chances in a thousand of stroke; and all three, 171 chances in a thousand of a stroke![2]

There are other causes:

4. *Obesity* contributes to high blood pressure, heart disease, diabetes, and cancer. Recently, a federal panel of experts claimed that obesity has risen to epidemic proportions in America. And this is in the midst of the supposed fitness boom!

5. *Stress* and *tension* are described by over half of those severely disabled as a basic cause of their heart problems.

6. *Diabetes.* There is a close relationship between diabetes and heart disease, possibly related to elevated blood cholesterol and lipids associated with the diabetic.

7. *Age* and *gender.* The older one is, the greater the possibility of heart disease. Men are more susceptible than women, though with increased cigarette smoking and job-related stress, women are catching up!

8. *Heredity.*

9. *Physical inactivity* seems to make one more susceptible to many ills that the more active avoid. Aerobic exercise, which we will discuss later, strengthens the heart and keeps blood vessels open and functioning properly.[3]

This list of known causes contains the clues for treating oneself better. Later in this chapter, we will discuss more systematically the prevention, reversal, and treatment of these conditions.

Health and the Threat of Cancer

Cancer is the second largest killer, accounting for 19 percent of all deaths in the United States. Based on medical statistics, experts estimate that about one-third of all Americans will develop a malignancy (cancer) in their lifetime. At least one-half of these people will die from their malignancy.

Harris H. McIlwain and associates point out that it is difficult to identify the agents that cause cancer. This is because cancer usually does not develop after a single exposure to a carcinogen. Usually, there are many exposures over long periods of time. More years may elapse before the cancer becomes apparent. Further, once a possible cause is removed, it again takes years before there is a decrease of risk. They offer the example of the risk of lung cancer from smoke exposure. Very few persons develop cancer in less than twenty years of smoking. (Not all smokers develop lung cancer.) It takes seven to ten years after stopping smoking to gain an appreciable reduction in the risk of lung cancer.[4]

There are two things a person can do to counter the threat of cancer. One is to identify and remove as many as possible of the risk factors that may lead to cancer. Persons may wonder if this is possible. If one is to believe all the news reports, nearly everything is a cancer-causing agent! However, for the most part we will be wise to avoid those that are known carcinogens. The list includes at least the following:

1. *Smoking.* Compared to nonsmokers, smokers face nearly ten times the risk of developing lung cancer, plus increased risk of cancer of the larynx, mouth, throat, esophagus, bladder, and pancreas. Smoking is also a factor in heart and lung disease.
2. *Alcohol.* In combination with tobacco, alcohol increases risk of cancer in the mouth, throat, larynx, and esophagus.
3. *Radiation.*
4. *Chemicals.* Many industrial and medical chemicals have been identified as carcinogens. These are removed from use when discovered, but effects may linger.
5. *Hormone treatment.* Use of the female hormone estrogen has been connected with increased risk of cancer of the lining of the uterus. At the same time, there is evidence that synthetic estrogens may protect against development of osteoporosis. As with many medications, there is benefit and risk that should be discussed with one's physician.
6. *Exposure to sunlight,* without clothing or a sunscreen, increases the risk of developing certain skin cancers.
7. *Diet.* Studies show that one is wise to avoid obesity; decrease fat intake; eat more high-fiber foods such as whole-grain cereals, fruits, and vegetables; include foods rich in vitamins A and C; include cruciferous vegetables such as cabbage, broccoli, brussels sprouts, and cauliflower; and restrict the use of salt-cured, smoked, and nitrite-cured foods.[5]

The second thing one can do is to seek early detection of health problems. One way to do this is through regular physical examinations. A later section of this chapter will suggest the types and recommended frequency of exams.

Still another way is through self-exam and self-awareness. The American Cancer Society suggests seven warning signals of which to be aware.

1. Change in bowel or bladder habits.
2. A sore that does not heal.
3. Unusual bleeding or discharge.
4. Thickening or lump in breast or elsewhere.
5. Indigestion or difficulty in swallowing.
6. Obvious change in wart or mole.
7. Nagging cough or hoarseness.

Other Health and Aging Issues

We have spoken of the two major families of illness that present the largest number of health problems to middle-aged and older adults. There are, of course, other causes of death, such as accidents. Three percent of all deaths result from nonautomobile accidents, and 2.4 percent are from automobile-related accidents.

There are a number of health problems for middle-aged persons that are not quite so ominous, but they are present and "pesky." Let's take a look at some of the changes in the human body. We will also consider some of the risks that simply go with the process of adding years.

There are a number of exterior changes that occur to the body over the years. The skin begins to change. Some layers of skin become thinner with age, and thus may tear or bruise more readily. Changes in fibers and thickness of skin also mean that at points on the body skin becomes looser and wrinkled. These wrinkles may first be noticed on the face.

There is a slight change in height; people become a bit shorter. Some have estimated that there is an average loss of about 1.2 cm (less than half an inch) every twenty years after reaching maturity. Weight, on the other hand generally increases as adults mature. Generally, weight peaks at ages 40 to 60, then levels out at 65 to 75, then gradually declines.

Quite often the size of the abdomen gradually increases after ages 35 to 45. This is because the body starts storing more fat deposits in the abdomen, even though one's total weight may decline. Regular exercise can minimize this factor, but it will not entirely eliminate it.

On the other hand, some fatty tissue under the skin will decrease over the years, perhaps beginning at age 40 or 50. As a result, bony prominences—such as the spine, shoulder blades, facial bones, and bones of the chest—may become more apparent.

Hair may start becoming gray as early as one's twenties. Probably half of the population has graying of some hair by age fifty. Thinning of hair and hair loss is also quite common. Occasionally, new hair appears in some areas of the body. None of these are a sign of anything but normal aging process.

For the teeth, concern shifts from cavity prevention to prevention of gum disease (periodontal disease). This may cause gum shrinkage, and cavities become more common at the roots of the teeth rather than the crown. Tooth enamel often becomes darker. Teeth position may shift. There is a gradual recession of gum tissues, but this can be slowed by good dental health practices.

There are also internal signs of aging. As we have noted, the heart and blood vessels undergo some changes. However, with normal health, one can expect to continue vigorous exercise even into old age. There may be a number of circulation problems. Some experience these in the feet and legs, revealed by swelling. This comes from a decreased return of blood and fluid from the feet, back toward the heart.

Muscles have become less elastic, resulting in more aches and pains and in slower recovery from such discomfort. By the time one reaches age forty, one's eyes will probably have increasing difficulty focusing up close. This is a normal aging change. Everyone usually suffers gradual decrease in their ability to hear sounds with increasing age.[6]

Gail Sheehy has noted a health issue that, sooner or later, every midlife woman will experience—menopause. She describes this process as the transition between a woman's reproductive state and a different internal hormonal milieu. It occurs gradually over a wide range of time, sometimes coming earlier than most people expect. Studies indicate that 10 to 15 percent of women seemingly come through this transition with no problems. Another 10 to 15 percent may be rendered temporarily dysfunctional. The rest—at least 70 percent of all women—wrestle with varying degrees of discomfort and with difficulties that come and go over a period of years. In response to the taboo of even discussing this topic, and because of the inadequacy of medical knowledge and assistance, she wrote *The Silent Passage*.[7] It provides a summary of known information and is a tool for further discussion and exploration of this topic.

I cannot prevent any of the various aspects of this aging process, though I can slow down some parts of it. Further, I can be vigorous and healthy while in the process of growing older.

Suggestions for Healthful Living in the Middle Years

The previous sections have contained many clues and indications of what shape healthful living should take in the adult years. At this point in life, we may be relatively symptom-free, or we may already be contending with one or more of the health problems mentioned above. Still, we can choose a manner of living that contributes to wholeness. Here are some suggestions.

EXERCISE—REGULARLY AND FAITHFULLY

Consistent exercise has a number of benefits. For one thing, it contributes to strengthening the lungs and vitalizing the cardiovascular system. A program of gradually increasing exercise has self-evident benefits: One is able to increase the amount of exercise and to feel better during and after the workout.

Another good result is that exercise contributes to weight loss. Exercise burns up calories that might otherwise go to body fat. Vigorous workouts also increase the rate of body metabolism (the process by which the body transforms food into energy and living tissue) for some hours after the workout.[8]

There is yet another vital result of good exercise practices. Such workouts can considerably decrease symptoms of depression. After a thorough study of the impact of exercise on psychological well-being, Dr. Robert S. Brown, a psychiatrist from the University of Virginia, concluded, "I've demonstrated to my satisfaction that not just exercise, but athletic-type training will reduce both anxiety and depression at the highly significant level statistically."

Dr. Thaddeus Kostrubala, author of *The Joy of Running*, agrees. He writes, "I have talked to many runners—runners who run long, medium, and short distances—and I have come to the conclusion that running done in a particular way is a form of natural psychotherapy. It stimulates the unconscious and is a powerful catalyst to the individual psyche."[9]

Runners speak of the "runner's high," a sense of euphoria that sometimes comes in the middle of a workout. They also comment on decreased tension, a relaxed approach to problems, and more focused attention to issues before them after the run.

The type of exercise that brings these benefits is, for the most part, aerobic exercise. This simply means exercise in which the muscles burn oxygen while using nutrients as fuel sources. By contrast, there is "anaerobic exercise," in which the muscles use glycogen (glucose) as the fuel source without burning oxygen. In aerobic exercise, one's heart rate is moderately elevated and breathing is somewhat heavier, but the person is able to talk while working out.

Running is the most popular form of aerobic exercise, but there are many others—brisk walking, swimming, water aerobics, cross-country skiing, racket sports (if you keep moving), biking, games that require continuous running and movement, and aerobic dance, to mention a few.[10] Benyo and Provost suggest the following guidelines for developing an exercise program:

1. View your pursuit of fitness as *fun* and not as work.
2. Perceive your physical activity as *play* and not as exercise.
3. Work out a minimum of three times a week for twenty minutes minimum. Five times a week for thirty minutes is ideal.
4. Be patient—set realistic, attainable goals. Map out a year-long program.
5. If your life is otherwise stressful, use your "play" time to *relieve* stress, not create more.
6. Abide by the hard/easy principle. Remember the formula of Stress + Rest = Performance (that is, increased physical skill and stamina).
7. Maintain a positive attitude about your workouts. Remember, any new or increased aerobic activity you do now is more than you were doing yesterday. Adjust your expectations accordingly.[11]

DEVELOP AND MAINTAIN A HEALTHFUL DIET

Good nutrition can aid in preventing many diseases and in enhancing one's vigor. Dietary habits figure in five of the nation's ten leading causes of death, including cancer, stroke, heart disease, diabetes, and atherosclerosis.

If one is struggling with high blood pressure, there are several dietary steps one can take to reduce the problem. These include:

- Adopt nutritionally sound eating habits, meeting the basic daily requirements of vitamins, minerals, proteins, roughage, fats, and carbohydrates.
- Eliminate or greatly reduce consumption of tobacco, alcohol, and caffeine.
- Radically decrease salt intake.
- Exercise, weight reduction, and efforts to control stress and anxiety.[12]

Recently, preliminary information from a massive study of nutrition in China was released. Dr. T. Colin Campbell was the American researcher associated with this project. In this research endeavor, 6,500 Chinese persons in a variety of settings each contributed 367 facts about their eating and other habits. While many implications are still being researched, several important conclusions may be noted. Jane Brody reports some of these findings:

> Reducing dietary fat to less than 30 percent of calories, as is currently recommended for Americans, may not be enough to curb the risk of heart disease and cancer. To make a significant impact, the Chinese data imply, a maximum of 20 percent of calories from fat—and preferably only 15 to 20 percent—should be consumed.
>
> Eating a lot of protein, especially animal protein, is also linked to chronic disease. Americans consume a third more protein than the Chinese do, and 70 percent of American protein comes from animals; only 7 percent of Chinese protein does. Those Chinese who eat the most protein, especially the most animal protein, also have the highest rates of such "diseases of affluence" as heart disease, cancer, and diabetes.[13]

Dr. Campbell concludes, "We're basically a vegetarian species and should be eating a wide variety of plant foods and minimizing our intake of animal foods."[14]

Cory SerVaas, M.D., suggests the following dietary guidelines as health-wise. They are supported by the early results of the Chinese study.

Choose More Often

Peas and beans:
- Pinto, black, kidney, garbanzo, navy, white, and lima beans; lentils; black-eyed and split peas

Low-fat or skim-milk dairy products:
- Low-fat or skim milk and buttermilk
- Low-fat yogurt
- Evaporated skimmed milk, nonfat dry milk
- Low-fat cheese (ricotta, pot, farmer or cottage, mozzarella, or cheeses made from skim milk)
- Sherbet, frozen low-fat yogurt, ice milk

Fats and oils:
- "Diet" and low-fat salad dressings
- Low-fat margarine

Lower-fat poultry, fish, and meat:
- Chicken, turkey, Rock Cornish hens (without the skin)
- Fresh and frozen water-packed canned fish and shellfish

Snack foods:
- Fruits and vegetables
- Breads and cereals

Cruciferous vegetables:
- Choose several servings each week. Brussels sprouts, cabbage, broccoli, cauliflower, rutabagas, turnips.

Food preparation:
- Baking, oven broiling, boiling, stewing (skimming off fat), poaching, stir-frying, simmering, steaming
- Use nonstick cookware to avoid extra fat.
- Season vegetables with herbs, spices, or lemon juice

Choose Less Often

Higher-fat poultry, fish, and meat:
- Duck and goose
- Poultry with skin
- Frozen fish sticks, tuna packed in oil
- Regular luncheon meats, sausage
- Beef, veal, lamb, and pork cuts with marbling, untrimmed of fat

Full-fat dairy products:
- Whole milk
- Butter
- Yogurt made from whole milk
- Sweet cream, sour cream, half-and-half, whipped cream, other creamy toppings (including imitation)
- Cream cheese, cheese spreads, Camembert, Brie

- Hard cheeses such as cheddar, Swiss, bleu, American, Monterey Jack, Parmesan
- Ice cream
- Coffee creamers (including nondairy)
- Cream sauces, cream soups

Fats and oils:
- Vegetable and salad oils, shortening, lard, meat fats, bacon
- Mayonnaise and salad dressings
- Gravies, butter sauces

Snack and bakery foods:
- Donuts, pies, pastries, cakes, cookies, brownies
- Potato chips and snack crackers
- Canned puddings, icings, candies made with butter, chocolate
- Granola, croissants

Food preparations to avoid:
- Batter and deep-fat frying, sautéing
- Use of fatty gravies and sauces
- Adding cream or butter to vegetables[15]

Some of us may have had healthy eating habits for years. If so, we face little or no change in adopting such a lifestyle. But many of us have not been making good food choices, and so we have many changes—in attitude and food selection—to make.

I am one of the latter group. For years, eating has been a form of entertainment, one I enjoyed very much. I grew up in beef-raising country, and a favorite meal was a huge portion of steak or a large hamburger, accompanied by something deep-fried. The meal would conclude with an equally large dessert.

For the last several months, I have been participating in a weight-loss program based on good basic nutrition. As I have struggled with making these changes in my life, I have discovered, at least for myself, some important things. I have learned that I can still enjoy eating as one of my forms of recreation, but perhaps it should not have as central a place as it once did. Other forms of gratification and reward should supplement eating.

When I have eaten *what* and *how much* I should have for the previous meal and have not snacked in between, there is a pleasant surprise. I am hungry and eager for the next meal. I will enjoy it, no matter what it is (with a few exceptions)!

Further, there is a delicious variety available within a nutritionally sound food plan. These foods can be enhanced with a number of herbs and spices. I can find something that fits my need in almost any restaurant, so I am wise not to forsake the delightful meals with friends I enjoy so much.

My mentors in this food plan point out that it is not a matter of eliminating foods I enjoy. Rather, my task is reducing how often and how much of them I eat. When I come back to one of these foods on the "less approved" list, either of two things happens: I may discover that I enjoy it even more as a rare treat; or I may discover that I am losing my taste for it. With a little more discipline, I discover something else: A taste of some rich foods is satisfying without consuming a whole portion. The first taste of a scrumptious dessert is really the best taste. I can share a dessert with someone. A bite or two of cheesecake or of hot fudge sundae can give me the experience, but few of the calories.

These are some of the steps I am taking toward better nutrition, which is so vital for one's present and future vigor and health.

ATTAIN AND MAINTAIN WEIGHT CONTROL

Nearly two-thirds of U.S. adults are overweight, according to a recent survey. This extra weight is a problem for a number of reasons. People don't look or feel their best when they carry extra pounds. More significantly, being overweight increases the risk of heart disease; diabetes; high blood pressure; gallstones; rectal, colon, breast, and prostrate cancers; and postsurgical complications.[16]

Quite probably, most of us have set out to lose weight and have found it difficult and very slow. The weight came on gradually, over the years. There are 3,500 calories in a pound of stored fat. So someone who ate ten more calories each day than his or her body used would gain a pound each year. (Ten calories is 1/5 of a fig newton or 1/54 of a Big Mac.)

Our body metabolism slows down when, as adults, we are no longer physically growing and maturing. I am told that, on the average, one's body needs 10 percent less food each subsequent decade after the age of eighteen. There is another characteristic of body metabolism that makes it difficult to lose weight. Over the centuries the human body has learned to adapt to droughts, food deprivation, and starvation. It does so by slowing down the metabolism so as to consume available body fat reserves much more slowly. (Thus does a person survive for a longer period during deprivation.) This same mechanism occurs in many diets. If there is a sudden change in the amount of food the body takes in, it responds by slowing the metabolism to match the amount of food available. This leads to a commonsense formula that has worked for many:

Sensible eating + moderate exercise = weight control

Sensible eating may include modest cutting back of one's intake. A reasonable plan is to decrease one's intake by no more than 500 calories a day. Matching exercise might ultimately be two and one-half miles of continuous walking or jogging (or some parallel activity as indicated above), four to five times a week. Then, be patient. Give it at least three months.[17]

There is another angle on weight loss from the China study mentioned earlier. These findings indicate that obesity is as much related to *what* people eat as it is to *how much*. Adjusted for height, Chinese people consume 20 percent more calories than Americans do. Yet Americans are 25 percent fatter. The main difference is in what is eaten. Chinese eat only one-third the amount of fat that Americans consume, but they eat twice the starch. Quite likely, the body stores fat but expends a larger proportion of carbohydrates. We should be aware of such findings as we start on our weight loss program.[18]

In speaking of obesity and weight loss, I am not implying that all middle-aged adults should be the same size and shape. It is cruel to impose over-thin expectations on either women or men. Whether within my weight goal or a bit beyond it, I have something of a "teddy bear" appearance, and I love it. People want to hug me! I have no intention of changing that, but I will monitor my weight on behalf of my health, vigor, and longevity.

FIND A PHYSICIAN YOU TRUST

Form a health-partnership with a physician you trust. Schedule appropriate exams at fitting times—with shorter intervals as you move through your middle years.

Too many of us avoid the doctor's office so long that we are not sure whom to call when an illness occurs. In the middle years, it is important to change this. Locate a doctor who has time for you, is interested in you, will work with you on your health issues.

Since early detection and prevention are keys to health in the middle years, you will need a range of examinations. Harris McIlwain and associates suggest the following to provide early detection of any cancer problems:

EARLY CANCER DETECTION[19]

Women

Breast examination	Every 2–3 years up to age 40, then yearly by a physician
Pelvic examination	Every 2 years after age 20 until age 40, then yearly
Pap test	By age 18, then every 2 years until age 70, then every 3 years
Mammogram	By age 38, then every 2 years to age 50, then yearly

Men and Women

Rectal examination	By age 30, then at age 35, age 40, then yearly
Stool test for blood	At age 40, then yearly
Sigmoidoscopy	This is a direct examination of the rectum and the adjacent area of the lower intestine. Recommended by some experts at age 50, then every 5 years. Some persons may need

	this more or less often. Ask your physician for advice on your own situation.
Skin changes	Watch your skin for new moles or old ones that change. If any area of skin becomes darker, new or old moles enlarge or bleed or become painful, see your physician.
Mouth and throat	Report any sores or color changes in your mouth that persist or are painful. This is especially important for persons who use *any* form of tobacco

Other Exams

Eye examination	Every 2 years
Dental examination	Yearly

There will be yet other examinations for the heart and other body systems. Consult with your doctor to see what exams are needed and at what frequency for the prevention, detection, and early treatment of any problems.

NEITHER UNDERUSE NOR OVERUSE MEDICATION

Some of us on the older end of middle adulthood were raised to believe "doctor knows best." We were to trust, believe, and explicitly obey what the doctor decided and said.

Without eroding respect for physicians, I am advocating a more active approach to health and medical issues. In selecting a doctor and in selecting a treatment for any health problem I have, I want to be a partner. If there are options for treatment, I'd like to know the other possibilities and why the doctor suggests the one she or he does.

In the past year, I have been under a doctor's care for a flare-up of a blood pressure problem. He prescribed a medication that promptly brought the blood pressure under control but had an unpleasant side effect. In turn, medication and treatment were prescribed for this side effect.

When I asked about the possibility of managing the blood pressure problem through lifestyle changes rather than medication, the doctor responded, "I encourage you on that. That's certainly to be preferred. However, most people want the quick fix when they bring me a problem."

The three currently best-selling prescription drugs are Tagamet, Inderal, and Valium, which are chemical treatments for ulcers, high blood pressure, and anxiety, respectively. These drugs only treat the symptoms; they do not address the causes. Indeed, they *mask* the causes. Nor do they cure the problems that brought about these health issues.[20]

Each of us needs to be clear how large a lifestyle adjustment we are willing to make. Then, in partnership with our physician, we will decide what medications are urgently needed, and which have benefits that outweigh their disadvantages. Then we will seek for ways to reduce or eliminate the medication by a healthy way of living.

ELIMINATE LIFE-THREATENING HABITS

One life-threatening habit is the use of tobacco. Throughout this chapter, cigarette smoking has been thoroughly indicted from every angle. While smokers speak of a few pleasures from smoking, the damage is immense. It is estimated that there are 300,000 tobacco-related deaths a year in this country. Some of these deaths, particularly those from lung cancer and emphysema, are often drawn-out, painful, and agonizing, both for the person dying and for loving persons gathered around.

This is another habit that is terribly hard to break. Fortunately, hospitals and other health organizations are offering methods and support groups to help. For starters, Tom Monte offers these guidelines:

- Set a target date. Give yourself reminders about this date. On the appointed date, throw all tobacco products away.
- Take up a sport. Exercise, rather than tobacco, can give one a lift.
- Examine your motives. Each time you pick up a cigarette ask yourself if you really want it.

- Consider nicotine spray. A doctor-prescribed, self-administered nicotine nasal spray has been found to reduce the craving for smoking.
- Try nicotine gum. Some studies show that half the people who use the gum are able to stop smoking.
- Use a nicotine patch. Some find this helpful in conjunction with other stop-smoking measures.
- Let your fingers do the walking. Your local chapter of the American Cancer Society or the American Lung Association may know of helpful programs, including counseling, relaxation training, hypnosis, or some other form of behavioral therapy.
- Go cold turkey. Eighty-five percent of former smokers preferred to stop all at once with no aids.[21]

For some, the use of alcohol may be another life threatening habit that should be confronted. I am not suggesting that moderate drinkers need consider it a problem. There is some medical indication that moderate drinking may have some beneficial effects. It may increase the amount of high-density lipoprotein in the body's blood, which in turn decreases the negative effects of cholesterol. Moderate consumption may be of help in calming highly stressed people, promoting recuperation. Moderate use might lead to a lower risk of hypertension. One researcher notes, "It is possible to conclude that a single nightly cocktail [or a glass of wine] might actually be therapeutic, but anything in excess of that could be detrimental to your health."[22]

As we have noted, the use of alcohol is a health problem when combined with smoking. This combination increases the risk for a number of cancers.

Alcohol consumption is a problem when it is overdone. Some people become morose, some violent, some humorous and entertaining. Speech is slurred, reflexes slow down, thinking becomes dull, and there is loss of memory. Beyond that, if a person continues drinking, she or he may become stuporous, or may black out and become comatose. If a person in any of these states attempts to operate a car, that person is life-threatening.

Alcohol consumption is also a problem if it leads to alcoholism. This is the continuation of uncontrolled drinking in spite of painful and harmful consequences to oneself and to others. Unfortunately we may not recognize alcoholism in ourselves, nor may those close to us. If there is any question at all, one should initiate a conversation with a physician, a counselor, or a member of Alcoholics Anonymous. If you are concerned that someone you care about may be an alcoholic, contact Al-Anon. Attendance at their meetings may clarify your concern and help you discover helpful strategies for coping and dealing with the problem.

I have already said that food consumption habits may need re-examination. For some, there may also be a need to reconsider the use of so-called recreational drugs. These might include marijuana, hallucinogens, stimulants, depressants, and narcotics. Many of these drugs must be illegally obtained, and this encourages drug trafficking in our country. Abuse of these substances can sneak up on a person if use has extended over the years. One is addicted when the necessity of drug use seriously interferes with health, work, or social functioning.[23] Fortunately, there are treatment programs and twelve-step programs, similar to Alcoholics Anonymous, for these problems.

It would be wise to look at our habits and ask if any are life-threatening, or if they are decreasing the quality of life for ourselves and for those around us.

Up to this point, my suggestions have focused mostly on the physical aspects of health. The following suggestions offer a broader perspective. As Scott Peck has noted, a person is a psycho-socio-spiritual-somatic being. Every illness has all of those aspects. So does health.

CULTIVATE LAUGHTER IN YOUR LIFE

Dr. Bernie Siegel fondly recalls Julie. She was a young woman who came to one of his support groups because of blindness due to diabetes. Julie had the gift of laughter and taught others in the group how this quality can make life better. Once, at a restaurant with family and friends, she was seated in a chair. Presuming the table was in front of her, she inched her chair forward. She continued to do so until she wound up across the room at the table of strangers. They asked, "Would you like to join us?" Julie exploded with laughter and was joined by everyone in the restaurant.

On another occasion, she was walking with her boyfriend, who was constantly and solicitously guiding her. He was so concerned, he fell off a curb. At this, she handed him her walking cane for the blind. "Here," she said, "take this. You need it more than I do." Julie has since regained her sight. Her comment out of this experience was, "Blindness taught me to see, and death taught me to live." Bernie Siegel would add that laughter taught her and others how to live life hopefully.[24]

Dostoevski once wrote, "If you wish to glimpse inside a human soul and get to know a man, don't bother analyzing his ways of being silent, of talking, of weeping, or seeing how much he is moved by noble ideas; you'll get better results if you just watch him laugh. If he laughs well, he's a good man. . . . I especially recommend it to the attention of young would-be brides. . . . All I claim is that laughter is the most reliable gauge of human nature. Look at children, for instance. Children are the only human creatures to produce perfect laughter, and that's just what makes them so enchanting."[25]

There are a number of health benefits that come from hearty laughter. Dr. Marvin E. Herring notes one when he comments, "The diaphragm, thorax, abdomen, heart, lungs, and even the liver are given a massage during a hearty laugh."[26] Norman Cousins had called this "internal jogging."

Humor also can jolt us out of habitual ways of thinking and can promote new perspectives. A sign of mental health is the ability to laugh at oneself in a gentle, mocking way. It is a sign that one has gained a larger perspective on the issue at hand.

There is also reason to believe that laughter activates the release of endorphins, the body's own pain-reducing substance. Endorphins also act as a stimulant to the body's immune system.[27]

So, then, for many reasons, one is wise to cultivate laughter in one's life. Find the things that bring a chuckle or a guffaw to your life. Read the comics, watch videos, listen to tapes, swap funny books, spend time with people who amuse you and bring out your playful side. It's good for your health.

At the end of each day, I have a few moments of quiet play awaiting me. For one thing, I spend a few moments reading the bridge column in the daily newspaper—having saved it until that time. Then, just before drifting off to sleep, I read an essay or two from a favorite humorist or storyteller. Some of my favorites are Erma Bombeck, Dave Barry, Robert Fulghum, Garrison Keillor, and Patrick McManus. In a life with many pressures, it is a relaxing, joyful way to end the day.

Laughter is a part of a larger topic, namely happiness and joy. It is perhaps the first step into that vast domain of which we shall speak more in a later chapter. We are health-wise when we remember and heed the practical wisdom of Proverbs 17:22, "A cheerful heart is a good medicine, but a downcast spirit dries up the bones."

RECOGNIZE, MANAGE, AND REDUCE THE STRESS IN YOUR LIFE

Stress is a topic so widely discussed that it may seem barely to need mention. However, we *know* more about stress than we *do* about it. Perhaps we know a lot about stress in general, but we do not always recognize its presence in our lives. We may not be aware how profound is its impact on health. So let's review a few health facts about stress and then sketch out a broad outline of healthy stress management.

From the work of Dr. Thomas H. Holmes and Dr. T. Stephenson Holmes, we are aware that stress can cause illness. Their work assigned "stress points" to a number of events, large and small, that bring stress to one's life. Major ones included death of a loved one, divorce, major illness or surgery, job change, or geographic move. One may have coping mechanisms for those major events, but there may be greater stress—and thus more health risk—from everyday hassles. These might include such matters as traffic tie-ups, misplacing things, noise, and having more things to do than there is time for.[28] One is less likely to have strategies for coping with those smaller irritations, which can accumulate.

Nor have we adjusted to the stress impact on our lives that comes from sensory overload in our lives today. Every major crisis and tragedy in the world is brought into our living rooms while it is in the process of happening. This contributes to the stress load we carry.

We have learned from pioneer Hans Selye about the General Adaptation Syndrome—the basic response to any stressor. This includes three stages: an alarm reaction, a stage of resistance, and then a stage of exhaustion. If this mechanism is called into play too frequently over the years, it can cause wear and tear on the body, including the breakdown of the immune system.

Stress may come from the stimuli outside us or from our internal responses. Our perception, self-expectation, jealousy, or inability to cope can make our response to stress much more powerful than one might first suspect.

We know that the complete absence of stress is neither desirable or possible. Stress may be good for us (sometimes called "eustress") if it stimulates and stretches our capacities. But stress is bad for us (then called "distress") when it impairs our mental outlook, makes us feel overwhelmed, and increases our susceptibility to physical disease.

Quite likely, none of us realize how much stress impact we are carrying within our personal health system until symptoms appear. It is known that continuous accumulated stress will impact one's more vulnerable organs, and then illness of that organ may develop. Some physical expressions of such stress include ulcers, high blood pressure, heart disease, menstrual disorders for women, impotence in men, gastritis, bladder trouble, asthma, headaches, allergies, and colitis.

Clearly a wise health policy is to recognize as many stressors as one can, then eliminate those one can and manage well those that cannot be eliminated. How can one do that? Here are a few beginning steps.

Reorder your priorities. Recognize what is most important in your life. Many middle adults try to juggle a much too heavy load. Career, marriage and parenthood, care of aging parents, plus some possible volunteerism and continuing education overcrowd our lives. It may all work when things are going well, but every one of those responsibilities may well have crises or tragedies within them at times.

It is wise to stop and ask, "Deep within me, what is my life about? What is most basic, most central, most important? What present needs should be at the top of my priorities? Do I need to simplify? If so, what can I let go of at this time of life?" In midlife, we ask these good questions with greater urgency.

Recognize the "small stuff." Dr. Robert Eliot, a cardiologist, has offered this advice: "Rule number one is don't sweat the small stuff. Rule number two is that it is all small stuff. And if you can't fight or flee, flow."[29]

Take a look at "flow" in your life. Is there an open channel, so that feelings and frustrations may dissipate soon after occurring? Or is the channel blocked, so that they become a huge dam of frustration, bursting once in a while with disastrous results? If so, perhaps you should ask a counselor or a trusted friend to help you find a different way. Accumulated anger and resentment only waste precious energy and give your body more with which to cope. Frustration or disappointment can lead either to redirection or to inner tenseness and problems. Recognize what is unimportant. Learn to live with the "flow."[30]

Develop explicit methods of stress management. Some of these might be quite simple. The only change might be to recognize how important they are. Then one can be sure that they are pursued often enough and long enough to help.

We have already spoken of physical exercise and of laughter as two such strategies. Time spent with deep, honest, and energizing friendships and with support groups can be another. Perhaps relaxing with music you enjoy will be helpful to you. A new hobby or fascinating activity might help you gain distance and perspective on your stress issues.

Attention has also been given to more explicit strategies for stress reduction. Harvard cardiologist Herbert Benson offered one such strategy. He studied the simplified version of Eastern meditation known as transcendental meditation. Out of that, he identified four elements in what he called the Relaxation Response. These are: (1) a quiet place with few distractions; (2) a comfortable position; (3) a passive and receptive attitude, which will allow thoughts to come and go without any effort to stop or control them; and (4) a "mantra"—a word, thought, or sound one repeats quietly to direct one's mind away from any conscious, distracting thoughts. Benson suggests that these four elements be brought together in two twenty-minute sessions each day. When that is done, he found, stress levels decrease.

Yet another form of relaxation is called biofeedback. By means of machines that monitor body temperature, muscular tension, and blood pressure, a person becomes aware of what is happening in his or her body. Then the person can learn how to lower blood pressure, relax muscles, and lower the body temperature. Through this technique, involuntary body responses can be brought under the control of the conscious mind.

Lloyd Ogilvie has noted that these findings point to an important insight. A quiet time each day can combat stress, change our attitudes, and transform our lives. The body needs that. However, this time can be an open door to an even greater peace-giving experience. This leads Ogilvie to suggest a second strategy, one more explicitly related to the Christian perspective. Using these methods, one can move into meditational prayer. One's "mantra" may be a statement of faith in one's Creator and Re-creator. One makes part of that quiet, relaxing time such a prayer as this: "God, speak to me. I'm listening. Use the process of my thoughts to say what I need to hear, understand, do. I yield my thinking brain to you."

One of the groups with which Ogilvie worked went on to create a confessional covenant that makes clear its individual and united efforts to manage stress. They call it "Ten Things I Will Do to Realize the Lord's Healing of Stress."

1. I recognize that stress is a major problem in my life.
2. I praise the Lord for the magnificent stress-coping mechanism [God] has given me.

3. I acknowledge the linkage between my thinking and attitudes and my body's stress-producing systems.

4. I am thankful that my body can produce eustress to assist me in meeting life's demands, challenges, and opportunities.

5. I seek to yield my thinking brain to the conditioning and control of the indwelling Christ.

6. I will set aside a time each day for meditation so that Christ can guide my thoughts and attitudes, decisions and actions, relationships and responsibilities.

7. I will quickly admit my inadequacy to manage stress and will talk to trusted confidants, fellow stress-strugglers, to release the build-up of stress, and receive from them encouragement and prayer.

8. I will meet consistently with my small group and seek to be as honest as I can be about how stress is affecting my life and what my attitudes may be doing to cause it.

9. I will pray daily for other members of the group, claiming Christ's healing power for them.

10. I will be sensitive to the things I do and say that cause stress in the people of my life and will, whenever possible, work to bring changes in the institutions, organizations, and groups of which I am a part to diffuse the stress-inducing society in America today.[31]

ADDRESS THE INTERFACE BETWEEN YOUR ENVIRONMENT AND YOUR HEALTH

Health is not a private, individual matter. Each of us lives in an environment that will either enhance our health or contribute to its deterioration. Each of us does well to ask, "What am I doing to my environment? What is my environment doing to me?"

There are a number of health hazards that occur because of growing populations, urbanization, and increased technology. Each of us may want to reflect on what impact such things as water, air, noise, traffic, food and drink, population, information, and hazardous waste pollution may be having on us.

A decision to improve one's health strategy may call for some decisions about environment. One can control a few of these personally, such as drinking bottled water or eating more fresh and less processed food. Others can be addressed in reasonably small social units—such as smoke-free environments at home or work. Many will need a societal response. The complexity and vastness of the needed response should not keep one from awareness and involvement. An increasingly poisoned environment would make good health impossible for anyone, so attention to one's environment is a significant health step.

RENEW GRATITUDE AND REVERENCE FOR THE GIFT OF LIFE

The final suggestion is a broad and important one. Its truth and significance is most often seen in its absence. Dr. Granger Westberg, founder of many Holistic Health Care Centers, believes that the illnesses of one-half to three-fourths of all patients originate in problems of the spirit. In his terms, physical symptoms are simply "tickets of admission" to a process of self-discovery and spiritual change.[32]

Dr. Carl Simonton and Stefanie Matthews-Simonton have noted there may be a cancer-prone personality. There may be certain combinations of traits that make some people particularly vulnerable to cancer. They list these: "First, a great tendency to hold resentment and marked inability to forgive; second, a tendency to self-pity; third, a poor ability to develop and maintain meaningful long-term relationships; and fourth, a very poor self-image."[33]

To help patients explore their emotions as a means to broad-based healing, Dr. Bernie Siegel asks persons four questions:

1. Do you want to live to be a hundred?
2. What happened to you in the year or two before your illness?
3. What does the illness mean to you?
4. Why did you need the illness?"[34]

Each of these noted healers point to a sweeping truth—that health or illness is part of the whole person, including one's attitude about one's life. Therefore, a decision for health includes steps in this area of one's life. Some of the pieces may be:

A decision to relate. Dr. James Lynch is absolutely convinced that loneliness is the number-one killer in the United States today.

Each of us may want to take stock of our loneliness. If we live alone, we may want to find intentional relationships with individuals or groups. If we are married and/or family and/or other committed relationships, we may want to identify the loneliness we feel in that relationship and seek a greater harmony. In a highly mobile, often distrustful, frequently competitive world, at least a few nurturing relationships are absolutely vital to one's health.

A decision to be self-honest. Bruce Larson tells of a retreat in which he participated. The central question at that gathering was, "Have you quit blaming others for your problems?" Such a question has a double thrust. It can lead one to discover that I alone have autonomy over my life and my emotions. No one can make me angry or depressed. Only I can choose that response, or another. It also leads to the question of forgiveness. If someone has wronged me, can I let it go, so it is not a barrier to my progress or to that relationship?

Carl Rogers once noted that there was only one kind of counselee that he considered relatively hopeless. That was the person who blames other people for one's problems. He pointed out that if you can own the mess you are in, there is hope and help available. As long as you blame others, you will be a victim the rest of your life.[35]

A decision to be vulnerable. On another journey, Bruce Larson noted a sign of life-changing importance. It was over the fireplace in a halfway house for emotionally disturbed people in western Ontario. The sign read, "Do you want to be right or well?" The sign was carefully chosen by the director. He was convinced that most persons with whom he worked needed to face that question. If one needs to justify one's every action and oneself in the eyes of others, not much progress could be made. To become well, persons needed to give up the illusion of always being right. Health begins when one can admit mistakes, needs, vulnerabilities. It starts when one can say, "Help!"

A decision to choose and treasure life. A most basic health question is, "Do I love and affirm life enough that I want to live better and longer?" Sadly, some people answer no. There may be guilt or suppressed rage and anger. Possibly, there are regrets or resentments about an unfulfilling life. A person may lack imagination or the will to see that there can be another way.

How much richer will be the life of someone who hears and believes Jesus' offer, "I came that they may have life and have it abundantly" (John 10:10). Then, perhaps we are ready to hear Moses' word to the people of Israel in Deuteronomy 30:19. "I call heaven and earth to witness against you today, that I have set before you life and death, blessing and curses; choose life, that you and your descendants may live."

In this chapter we have considered a vast range of issues on health in our midyears. These issues do not require that we add to life's agenda. They may require that we alter our routines of eating, drinking, exercising, thinking, feeling, relating, laughing, meditating, praying. We have been speaking of the interrelatedness of all of these aspects of our life. We have also been speaking of health as a spiritual concern.

John Pilch, spokesperson for the impact of spiritual values on wellness, says it well, "The key elements of wellness are knowing the purpose of life, understanding its genuine joys and pleasures, and assuming total and complete self-responsibility."[36] With such a perspective we are on the way to health and life, even in the middle of it.

For Personal or Group Reflection and Discussion

1. Take a look at the ten suggestions for health management. Do you agree with them? Do you feel that any are unnecessary for you? Would you add other suggestions?

2. How do you feel you are treating yourself in terms of your health? On which suggestions are you doing a good job? Where can you do better?

3. If you are exploring this book as a group, you might want to invite a physician, a nutritionist, and/or a physical fitness spe-

cialist in as a panel on health issues. What specifically would you like to ask them?

4. Upon what health practices would you like to make a covenant to do better? With whom would you like to make this covenant?

Resources

Benyo, Richard, and Rhonda Provost. *Feeling Fit in Your 40s*. New York: Atheneum, 1987.

Bostonia 52, no. 1 (winter 1978). Published by the office of Public Relations of Boston University.

Brody, Jane E. "China's Blockbuster Diet Study." *The Saturday Evening Post*, October 1990, 30–33.

Cousins, Norman. *Anatomy of an Illness as Perceived by the Patient*. New York: Bantam Books, 1979.

———. "The Laughter Prescription." *Saturday Evening Post*, October 1990, 34–39.

Eskin, Bernard A., and Lynne S. Dumas. *Midlife Can Wait: How to Stay Young and Healthy after 35*. New York: Ballantine Books, 1995.

Larson, Bruce. *There's a Lot More to Health Than Not Being Sick*. Waco, Tex.: Word Books, 1981.

McIlwain, Harris H., Lori F. Steinmeyer, Debra Fulghum Bruce, R. E. Fulgum, and Robert G. Bruce Jr. *The 50+ Wellness Program*. New York: John Wiley and Sons, 1990.

Monte, Tom. *Staying Young: How to Prevent, Slow, or Reverse More Than 60 Signs of Aging*. Emmaus, Pa.: Rodale Press, 1994.

Ogilvie, Lloyd. *Making Stress Work for You*. Waco, Tex.: Word Books, 1984.

Reisser, Paul C., Teri K. Reisser, and John Weldon. *New Age Medicine: A Christian Perspective on Holistic Health*. Chattanooga, Tenn.: Global Publishers, 1988.

Rowan, Robert L. *How to Control High Blood Pressure without Drugs*. New York: Charles Scribner's Sons, 1986.

SerVaas, Cory. "Diets That Protected against Cancers in China." *Saturday Evening Post*, October 1990, 26–29.

Sheehy, Gail. *The Silent Passage: Menopause*. New York: Random House, 1991.

Sherman, James R. *Middle Age Is Not a Disease*. Golden Valley, Minn.: Pathway Books, 1985.

Siegel, Bernie S. *Love, Medicine, and Miracles*. New York: Harper and Row, 1986.

3

Career
Decisions

RECENTLY, I LED a support group for job
hunters and career changers. Eight people par-
ticipated in the group, all of them in the middle third of life, all of
them previously or currently employed.

Five were unemployed job hunters.

- One, an early childhood specialist with a Ph.D., had been
  employed for twenty years in a prestigious private school. In
  spite of distinguished service, including faculty awards and ci-
  tations, she was dismissed by a new principal.
- Another was a university-trained middle manager with an insurance company. He was told after fifteen years of service
  that they were closing his department. When he offered to
  move, he was told no other opportunities existed.
- Still another had left a teaching position to move with her
  spouse, who wanted to pursue graduate education. She faced
  trying to find a new position in a less receptive environment.
  At the same time, she wondered if this was the time to explore
  something else.
- Yet another was attempting to begin a new career. Though
  previously employed in childhood education, she hoped to

work in her new field of expertise, supported by her recently earned master's degree in library science.

- The last one in this group had been putting much effort into obtaining clinical supervision credentials as an institutional chaplain. However, the accrediting committee had recommended that he not continue. This response almost surely closed the door on those aspirations. The time had come to consider other career options.

Three of the group were considering changing their careers. Of these three, two were nurses.

- One found her life, which combined single parenting with the demands of high-pressure cardiac-care nursing, was too demanding and out of control. She sought a career that would be more manageable and in accord with her other needs.
- The other, a mental health nurse, had entered this field because of the rich one-on-one care she could offer patients. Now, with the financial crunch and a shrinking patient population, her private hospital employer was abandoning that style for something more cost-effective. Her work was becoming unfulfilling to her.
- The third "career changer" was employed in the marketing research department of a major company. He told the group about the revolution taking place within the modern corporation. New styles of participant management, largely imported from Japanese examples, had altered the way decisions were made and work was done. This stimulated creativity, but also increased expectations and quotas. These higher expectations were in turn increased again the next year and the next. Along with greater productivity, there was much more work-related stress, from which he would like a change. Then, too, present tasks seemed somewhat distant from his growing interests in more personal expression and care. These were the topics that increasingly drew his interest and passion.

In many ways, this group epitomizes what had been happening to the world of work and to individual careers during midlife in recent years. Let's take a look at some of those changes in the workplace. Then I will describe the group's experience as we faced the issues before each of us.

Changes in the Work Marketplace

Carole Hyatt offers some perspectives in understanding today's employment marketplace. She suggests that the word to characterize these times is "contradiction." There is quick change, amidst the old. Those who adapt and learn, along with taking old skills into new places, are those most apt to succeed. She suggests that there are five critical factors in the marketplace.

The first is the globalization of business, which in turn brings influences from other cultures into the American workplace. As we noted above, Japanese management techniques are very much a part of American corporations. Persons and corporations from many parts of the world are both competitors with American business as well as investors in it and employers of American labor.

A second factor is rapidly expanding technological growth. Communications satellites, fax machines, and robotics are part of our present and future. So is advanced computer technology: The 6 million books in the Library of Congress can now be contained in computer storage devices that will fit into a five-by-seven-foot room.

Information technology is amazing and continually developing. American business will spend nearly $100 billion a year on data communication services alone. We live in the flowering of the Age of Information. Job opportunities in the high-tech computer fields are expected to grow massively, perhaps by 40 to 68 percent over the next few years.

Third, there is the restructuring of American business (and other institutions). Corporations may find reasons to merge, to add new services, or to close or sell off portions of the business. Any one of these changes may bring a large amount of job upheaval.

The employment pattern of corporations is also changing. In the 1970s and '80s, there was a tremendous growth of "middle manager" positions. Then, 2 *million* of them were fired, more because of the restructuring of business than for performance reasons.[1] This was the crunch the insurance person in our support group felt. As large numbers of early midlife "baby boomers" find themselves competing for these positions, there is a career squeeze, with less advancement, and even less pay increase. As Hyatt notes, "*Change*, not fairness, has always been the directional marker that business has chosen to follow. It's a hard truth to face, but it's the way it is."[2] In such changing times, all too often Jack Falvey's grim warning, "Performance has nothing to do with fate,"[3] is true.

Fourth, not only the corporation, but the worker's attitude, is changing. If there is less security, there is also less worker loyalty. One survey revealed a 60 percent decrease in employee loyalty over a five-year period.

All of this leads to the fifth factor, the wide diversity of career options. These options may emerge from development of new skills, finding new applications for existing skills, or from retraining and reeducation.

Increasingly, persons are finding their career opportunities in the small (and/or) new corporation or organization rather than the older and larger firms. Persons who started somewhere else are joining the fast-growing service part of our economy. Persons may work for themselves or for others out of their own homes.[4]

For the midlife person, other aspects of the employment picture need to be noted. One is the increased presence of both genders in virtually all employment areas. Further, many more midlife women are employed throughout their adult years, rather than entering the market at midlife, as was true for many in previous decades and generations.

All of this means that fewer and fewer of us will have the same or similar job titles with the same organization for all of our working lives. A few job titles are going out of existence. Many more are replacing them. Job titles of types of work have mushroomed to more than 45,000 known categories.[5] This is approximately double that of twenty years ago.

Each day, it is estimated that 80,000 persons join the ranks of job hunters, either by choice or necessity. Hyatt estimates that 12 million people are actively engaged in switching to a new career; 12 million more are planning to do so; and 25 million are contemplating such a change. The Rand Corporation projects that there will be twice this number of career changers by the year 2000. For now, one in five workers change jobs every year.

At present, the average person works at ten and one-half different jobs in a lifetime. There are at least three career changes in this average lifetime of work.[6] In this country, jobs now last an average of 3.6 years.[7] There may well be acceleration of these trends. Some estimate that within a decade or so, it will be a common occurrence for a person to have *six to ten* career changes over a lifetime!

Responding to Involuntary Job Loss

Many people make these changes because they lost their jobs. Expected or not, job loss carries a deep trauma. It may be because of a company squeeze or a negative performance evaluation. One may get one's termination notice alone or in the company of many others. There may be liberal severance benefits or practically none at all.

Whatever the circumstances, there is much that happens to one upon losing a job. Samuel N. Ray, who has helped many people deal with job loss, sees the following emotions frequently coming into play:

Denial. "It can't happen to me . . . It really didn't happen to me, did it?"

Shock. A person may experience physical symptoms, such as nausea, chills, fainting. People may be forcing decisions and actions on the person for which he or she is not ready.

Fear. There will be worries about finances, about facing friends, family, and colleagues and admitting what happened.

Loss of control. A regular job and paycheck gives one a sense of control over life. Now that is gone.

Anger. One may feel enraged over this injustice. There is a danger to take this out on family and friends, or to let it color one's views when searching and interviewing for new work. It needs to be ventilated, felt, experienced, and let go.

Hurt, rejection, humiliation. The anger may be turned inward, and if so, it may well attack one's self-understanding and self-esteem.

Guilt. There may be feelings of deserving the firing, of letting the family down, of failing to provide, of being unworthy of future employment.

Depression. This is a perfectly normal reaction to being fired. It is a frequent part of the response to shock, anger, hurt. If it lingers and affects one's ability to get back in the career search, then professional help should be sought.

Exhaustion. This may well include physical, mental, and emotional exhaustion, a deep bone weariness. A short rest and recovery time is certainly in order. After that, awareness of the problem of exhaustion, and establishing a balanced life—including diet, exercise, and job-hunting activities—is a fitting response.[8]

It is hard to overestimate the impact job loss has on a person's sense of well-being. Harry Brenner of Johns Hopkins University has noted that every 1 percent increase in unemployment brings a 2 percent increase in the nation's mortality rate, a 5 to 6 percent increase in homicides, a 5 percent increase in imprisonment, and a 3 to 4 percent increase in first admissions to psychiatric hospitals.[9]

Stephen Strasser and John Sena suggest a very specific strategy for responding to job loss.

1. *Walk away for a while.* Disengage from it for a brief time. Do not strategize, plan for the future, negotiate severance pay, request job references. Leave and get some rest and distance before discussing such matters.

2. *Accept the inevitable.* The employers have made a decision. There is nothing to be gained in arguing, cajoling, disputing, or expressing acrimony toward one's boss.

3. *If they'll let you resign, do it.* That is, if doing so does not adversely affect your unemployment insurance or severance package.
4. *Talk to supportive friends.* Find the persons who will listen, not give advice. Express all the anger, confusion, disbelief, conflicting emotions. These, they suggest, are all things that should be done on the first day.

For the next two days, one needs to gather all one's family, friends, and other support network persons, and express what one is feeling and experiencing. Strasser and Sena note:

> It is often vital to your psychological well being to vent your emotions and thoughts to another party. Do not, however, act on these emotions or thoughts. You may have the urge to call your boss and tell him you have seen better heads on glasses of beer. To tell your brother-in-law that you are now ready to go into his fertilizer business. To take out a loan so that you can buy a franchise specializing in yak milk (which is pink, by the way). RESIST ACTING ON THESE URGES.[10]

Hopefully, one gradually gains a bit of perspective. One may realize that others have gone through this and survived. There may be a bit of relief that instead of living in uncertainty one can now make specific plans. One can believe that there is another job out there that may be more rewarding than the last one.

These authors suggest that after the first 72 hours it's time to get on with your life. Now is the time to negotiate severance pay, job-hunting support services, recommendations, referrals, and suggestions from supervisors or colleagues.[11]

These experienced writers suggest a dynamic and decisive response to job loss. In all likelihood, not all will be able to respond this quickly. Those in our support group needed more time than that to absorb their loss. Still, the authors' advice is worthy. A crisis that may come fairly frequently in life calls for effective coping and responding skills. Even if the first steps are unsteady and faltering, they should be taken.

Options for the Voluntary Career Changer

In a chapter that is only partially tongue-in-cheek, humorist Dave Barry asks, "What triggers the male midlife crisis?"

Generally the midlife crisis is triggered when a male realizes one day at about 2:30 p.m. that he has apparently . . . devoted his entire life to doing something he hates. Let's say he's a lawyer. . . . He worked *hard* to become a lawyer. . . . And then one afternoon, while writing yet another deadly dull formal letter to a client, a letter filled with standardized, prefabricated phrases . . . he realizes that he hates *everything* about being a lawyer . . . his clients . . . other lawyers . . . the way every time he tells people what he does for a living, they react . . . his office . . . Latin phrases . . . his *briefcase*. . . . He decides he wants to have a *completely different* job, something fun, something carefree, something like . . . hang-gliding instructor.

Meanwhile, somewhere out there is a middle-aged hang-gliding instructor who has just discovered that he hates *his* life . . . not making enough money . . . sudden down drafts . . . having to be nice to vacationing lawyers . . . he wants . . . a better-paying job that enables him to do something truly *useful* with his life . . . a doctor.

Of course, if he did a little research, he'd find that most doctors hate the medical profession. They hate getting sued . . . the way everyone assumes that they're rich . . . their beepers . . . peering into other people's personal orifices. They wish they had a career with less responsibility . . . a *fun* career. . . . They wish they were: humor writers.

My point is that there's no reason for you to feel depressed about being trapped in Career Hell, because so is everyone else. Doesn't that make you feel better? No? Hey, look, at least *you* can put this book down. . . . *I* have to sit here and finish this stupid chapter so that I can meet my stupid deadline. . . . As soon as I finish the aforementioned chapter, I'm applying to law school.

Is there any proven method for coping with a midlife career crisis? If you put that question to a group of leading psychologists, they wouldn't bother to answer you. They're *sick* of dealing with your pathetic little problems. They want to be test pilots.[12]

Dave Barry suspects that the way to deal with this mid-career boredom and frustration is to have a secret identity. For example, when Bruce Wayne tires of being a wealthy millionaire, he can become—*Batman*! With more women participating in the workforce lifelong, there is a quite similar female midlife crisis. Quite likely there are similar fantasies to help one cope.

In today's turbulent, stress-filled work environment, it may be difficult to keep enthused and focused on one career throughout a working lifetime. Some of us may view the possibilities of change and variety with enthusiasm. There are a variety of choices and options facing us. Let's look at each of these in turn.

OPTIONS

Some of us may be *starting* a career path. Various reasons and decisions may have kept us out of the employed group until the middle third of life. A couple may have made a decision that only one be employed. There may have been choices to give home child care a priority for a time. A term of military service or extended education may mean that some persons come to the civilian workforce at this time of life. Those who do so have one advantage. They may have interest and enthusiasm beyond that of many contemporaries. There is also one disadvantage—others their age have experience and advance placements.

Some may be seeking *career renewal.* Many sense that they are in the right general area but need some personal revitalization within that career. This can come in a variety of ways. A person may identify specialties within the career where one really shines. Then one may polish those skills and seek ways that these specialties are emphasized. One may sense that one's present employment is stifling one's creativity. Either job change or renegotiation of job conditions might be helpful. Perhaps there are new developments that call for continuing education and exploration, which in turn help an old career feel new.

Some may want to engage in *career assessment, evaluation, and, very probably, career change.* Personalities do change over a lifetime. Some interests, some creative juices may get used up. The job or career itself may have changed so much that it no longer holds the appeal it once did. Every workplace has a few employees who have stayed there too long. Quite visibly, they find the work dull and boring, are given to cynicism, despair, self-pity. Persons who discover they are on the brink of falling into such traps—or have already done so—may need to look for a more complete change in career focus and direction.

In this connection, Tom Jackson suggests that for the growing person, today's rapidly changing work scene offers exciting possibilities. He urges, "Stay loose. . . . For the open mind there are open doors."[13] He points out that the growing, becoming person may qualify for careers that did not previously exist. For example, here are ten jobs that did not exist in the mainstream of employment ten years ago: (1) personal fitness coach, (2) Eurocurrency trader, (3) recycling consultant, (4) biogeneticist, (5) interactive video designer, (6) laser graphics expert, (7) wellness manager, (8) computer resume counselor, (9) video game designer, (10) Gray Panthers advocate.[14]

Not only may the widely experienced, broadly trained, imaginative person qualify for new careers, she or he may be able to help create previously nonexistent ones. This may come from putting together a unique combination of skills.

Some may need to seek *renewal in spite of one's career.* We may sense that because of other commitments, we are tied to a given job in a given place that holds few of the possibilities of which we have just spoken. Rather than fall into despair over such a situation, it may be wise to find other sources of personal renewal. Perhaps the relationships at work can be enhanced. Perhaps education and leisure in one's off-work hours can bring enrichment. Possibly a hobby, avocation, volunteer activity, or second job will provide the "spark." I will speak more on this shortly.

WORK STYLES

Along with a variety of options, there is a variety of work styles. Carole Hyatt introduces this concept and suggests that work style is a broad picture of how one interacts with others and the process of work itself. It includes how one visualizes possibilities and acts upon them, how one solves problems, and how one impacts one's organization.[15] She identifies four basic work styles. First, there is the *Lifer*.

> The Lifer . . . stands firm about where he or she belongs: *with one company* or in one profession, often for a lifetime. *Two* long term jobs—or one change of profession—is about their limit. Lifers are monogamous types, people who tend to find what they need in a single relationship—with a profession, a product, a company, or a talent, such as music or art. They are committed for the long run. This "long-term marriage" may not be perfect, but its foundation is strong, the familiarity is comforting, and it provides the sense of continuity much required by a Lifer.[16]

In order to achieve this continuity, the Lifer will be a gifted diplomat and learn to adjust to new managers or new owners. An abiding sense of connection to work is important. They are motivated, ambitious, and among the shrinking group of those fiercely loyal to an organization or profession. They want consistency. They work best in organizations where there is a presence of power, authority, and continuity.

Second, there is the *Builder*.

> Take the Lifer and introduce a *second*, or even a third vocation to which he/she is passionately committed and you have the Builder. Now think *parallel lives* and you get a sense of what the Builder is all about. The Builder, like the Lifer, seeks the foundation and security of the long-term commitment, but unlike the Lifer, the Builder is not content with a single marriage. His/her tendency is an honorable bigamy—the Builder has found another true love and will not relinquish the one he/she knows best for the one newly discovered.[17]

Builders have vital interests in their secondary careers. For example, a trial lawyer may perform with a jazz band on a semi-professional basis. The Builder knows clearly where his or her priorities lie. Yet, the Builder needs the second career-interest-passion to help him or her feel complete and to remain committed to the first and basic career.

Such folk are energetic achievers. They assume second identities after their first day's work is over. They see work as play, work as an extension of their spirit. This description fits me. While my primary career is as a pastor, my vigorous hobby is researching topics of interest to me, writing on them, leading seminars on them. At this very moment, I sit—after the end of a work day—enjoying the telling of this exploration.

Third, there is the *Synthesizer*.

The Synthesizer has some of the Builder's energy, some of the Lifer's inclinations toward security, but primarily, the Synthesizer is always alert to *opportunities*. Ever ready to hop on the next step Aup, a Synthesizer's career, were you to diagram it, develops the shape of an inverted pyramid, widening at the top as he/she learns . . . and does more.

Synthesizers have a combination of talents, skills, and work experience that increasingly makes them eminently promotable. . . . Synthesizers tend to accept change with greater ease and more confident risk takers. . . .

Many Synthesizers are successful late bloomers, finding their niche after four or five careers and many false starts.[18]

Synthesizers recognize and develop a wide variety of skills and see them like various ingredients for a recipe. Such persons are able to take what appears to be two or three diverse skills and combine them into something new and different. They are receptive to suggestions. Further, they are good at asking insightful questions, and are able catalysts. They are adaptive risk takers.[19]

Fourth, there is the *Reinventor*.

When one's situation calls for a new outlook, one may shift gears dramatically in thinking about one's career. With seeming radical discontinuity from what one has done before, one may change careers.

This requires courage, self-understanding, and *will*—and sometimes a disruption so serious that such a change must be considered. "Reinventors have a high tolerance for ambiguity and deal brilliantly with sudden crises or quick-change priorities. They prefer a looser kind of control."[20] They are also realists about what works and doesn't work for them.

These styles are not mutually exclusive. Nor is one tied to a single style for a lifetime. Personal preference or life circumstance may demand a change from one to another. But they are useful categories to help one understand one's preferable way of operating in the confusing maze of career choices.

Our Group's Process

Against this background I now report the process of the support group described at the beginning of this chapter. It is my hope that all job hunters and career changers will undertake this task in a group, even a group of two persons. There are several reasons for needing a group. Persons who have been there can offer sympathetic support for others who have lost their jobs. Further, job hunting is a lonely and often discouraging task! There are inevitable rejections in the search. And it's hard to get motivated to start. Other persons that both support each other in the pain and hold each other responsible for working at it can be a valuable gift. Such a group may be led by someone with some experience and expertise (this is probably preferable). Or it may be a group of people all struggling together, who report progress and reflect on ideas found in some of the books I suggest at the end of this chapter.

I am privileged to have been trained by Richard Bolles, author of the best-selling *What Color Is Your Parachute?*, in the eclectic process he describes in that book. Since my training, I have led hundreds of people in Life/Career Planning groups.

While I intended to use that knowledge to lead these people, I had a clear sense this particular group was unique. These persons had many years of successful experience behind them. They were deeply into career crises or transitions. They were an astute group—indeed, two of them had gone through a similar life/career planning process fifteen years before. Further, they were in a rather somber employment atmosphere. Not only was much of the workplace restructuring, they were in a down employment period. Seven percent unemployment rates were being reported.

The common theme was that each person in the group had experienced some sort of "trigger event" that launched that person into a time of change. For some, this was an inward "trigger"—interior messages about loss of enthusiasm or frustration with work. For some, the "triggers" were external—dismissal, divorce, or geographic moves. All of us had some "endings" to accept. We had to come to terms with those endings. Each person was in a "neutral zone," letting go of some old things and searching for some new ones. Even if such transitions happen fairly often in today's world, these times are still extremely uncomfortable. This discomfort contributed to an urgency and an openness with each other.

SUPPORT

We began by hearing each other's stories. Rather quickly, our stories drew us together. We had a clear sense that "We're in this together." We encouraged each other in disappointment and celebrated with each other in triumphs. We updated each other on our progress and held each other accountable for taking intended steps. From this, a group energy—greater than each individual's—became a part of our experience.

WHAT? WHERE?

Richard Bolles has suggested that the job hunt/career change task has three parts: (1) *What?* (2) *Where?* and (3) *How? What* particular skills do I have to offer? (These should be skills that I enjoy using.) *Where* do I want to use these skills? *How* do I locate that work opportunity and get myself hired *where* I can use *what* I have to offer? He suggests that too often the job hunter attempts to answer question three, the *how*, without adequate attention to the *what* and *where*. When this happens, the search is short-circuited. The person who conducts this search wisely will give attention to each of these aspects in turn.

Bolles often visualizes this process as a flower. He has placed the most crucial questions of self-knowledge for one's job hunt on various petals of this flower. Our group built on Bolles's wisdom and experience. Part of each session was given over to personal self-discovery as each person filled in the details on his or her personal flower.

The job hunters integrated these discoveries as they carried on their search for employment. Because of economic necessity, some of the job hunters did not have the luxury of waiting for all the results to be in. Still, they reported "aha!" moments of self-discovery as we carried on this investigation. These discoveries empowered them and helped them sort and evaluate possibilities that came their way.

THE PERSONAL FLOWER

The petals on the personal flower are:

1. Physical setting
2. Spiritual or emotional setting
3. My favorite skills
4. My favorite kinds of information
5. My favorite kinds of people
6. My favorite kinds of things
7. My favorite outcomes
8. Reward

Let's take a look at each petal.

Physical setting. This has two aspects: (1) Where in terms of geography would I like to do my work? If I must move to obtain employment, what geographical factors (for example, weather, recreation opportunities, services) are important to me? (2) What are the work conditions in which I am most effective? One might begin by asking the opposite—What distasteful work conditions would I like to avoid in my next and all future jobs? (We seem to remember those vividly!) Then translate them into positive conditions and rank them in order of importance.

Spiritual or emotional setting. What is my philosophy of life, and therefore, what needs to be true about my workplace? (For example, if I am committed to truth telling, can I be honest in my workplace?) What purposes, goals, and values would I like to serve with my life—including my employment?

For our group, this was a crucial issue. We came at this topic from a Christian perspective. The Bible speaks often about God's call to individuals and groups. Indeed, the term *vocation* comes from the Latin word *vocatio*, meaning "summons." We believe that God calls to persons from the needs of God's world. To hear that call and one's unique place in responding is a most basic part of life planning. Frederick Buechner says it well:

> There are all different kinds of voices calling you to all different kinds of work, and the problem is to find out which is the voice of God rather than that of society, say, or . . . self-interest. By and large a good rule for finding out is this: the kind of work God usually calls you to is the kind of work (a) that you need most to do and (b) the world most needs to have done. If you really get a kick out of your work, you've presumably met requirement (a), but if your work is writing TV deodorant commercials, the chances are you've missed requirement (b). On the other hand, if your work is being a doctor in a leper colony, you have probably met (b), but if most of the time you're bored and depressed by it, the chances are you haven't only bypassed (a) but probably aren't helping your patients much either. The place God calls you is the place where your deep gladness and the world's deep hunger meet.[21]

My favorite skills. My favorite skills are what I like to do with *Things*, *People*, and/or *Information*. One of the most exciting experiences in following this process is skill discovery and thus personal empowerment. Bolles has identified several erroneous but widely held ideas about skills. Overcoming these is the first step to skill identification and empowerment:

Erroneous idea one: *People are not born with skills. All skills must be acquired.* Not true. Many skills seem to be inborn.

Erroneous idea two: *Skills are acquired mostly at school.* The truth is that skills can be acquired almost anywhere—home, recreation, work, etc.

Erroneous idea three: *One will be aware of the skills one has.* Untrue. Some sort of skill identification is usually necessary.

Erroneous idea four: *Skills are not transferable from one field to another.* Again untrue. Many skills are readily transferable from one occupation to another.

Erroneous idea five: *I have just a few skills, probably unmarketable.* Untrue! Most people have 500 to 700 skills! These can be identified. The marketable combinations of those skills will likely be much larger than one imagines.[22]

To overcome these erroneous ideas and experience the exciting discovery of skills, our group gave a good bit of time to skill identification. Each person was asked to reflect over his or her life and identify several "satisfying accomplishments"—a task that a person did that gave a feeling of joy and accomplishment at the time. The person then wrote a simple description of that accomplishment. We then gathered in groups of three. In turn, each read his or her satisfying accomplishment and identified the skills used in it. The other two persons invariably located numerous other skills and reported those. These skills were then recorded on a chart provided in Bolles's *Quick Job-Hunting Map*. As this was repeated several times, a pattern of one's most characteristic skills, used *and enjoyed*, began to emerge.

As we engaged in this process, we were informed by the perspective that there are three families of skills. The first family is that of *functional* skills. These are the abilities one uses in acting on *people, information (or data)*, and *things*. These are akin to aptitudes. They exist across time—if one had them in childhood, one still has them—perhaps rusty, perhaps more sophisticated. These skills are so much a part of a person that one is often scarcely aware one has them. And they are readily transferable from one occupation to another.

The second family is *self-management* skills. This has to do with how one manages life, gets along with others, relates to space, impulses, etc. It includes humor, tact, sensitivity, promptness, ability to work under supervision or alone, openness to learn from criticism, etc. These are extremely important. More persons are hired because of them and fired because of lack of them (excepting the firings because of economic conditions, of course) than for any other reason. They are sometimes called "environmental skills," implying that one should locate the work environment where there is a good fit with the way one manages life. In the middle of the flower, one records information on both of these families of skills.

My favorite kinds of information. This brings us to the third family of skills. These are sometimes called *"special knowledge"* or *"work content"* skills, or simply *"information."* In these, one is using one's memory. These are the things one has learned. They are often thought of as the skills acquired in schools. However, such skills can be self-taught or learned on the job, in the home, from workshops or seminars, by observing others, by being mentored, or by reading. While these skills are often more specifically tied to one occupation, they also have applicability in other careers as well. In the fourth petal, one is invited to record both the content areas of one's information and the form in which one likes to engage it.

My favorite kinds of people. These are the people with whom I wish to use my skills. Again, there are two aspects. For one thing, what sort of people environment do I desire in my co-workers?

Important insights on people environments come from John Holland's perspective that there are six basic personality types. There are also six work environments—*R*ealistic, *I*nvestigative, *A*rtistic, *S*ocial, *E*nterprising, and *C*onventional. Actually each person is a combination of all six types in descending order, with perhaps three of the types being dominant. Each workplace also has these same characteristics, or a combination of them.

- *R*ealistic types are practical and prefer concrete tasks and problems. They prefer being outside, working with objects, machines, tools, plants, and animals.
- *I*nvestigative types are analytical and intellectual. They like to think through problems and like observing, investigating, evaluating, problem solving.
- *A*rtistic types are expressive, intuitive, and innovative. They like to express their selves through artistic media, using imagination and creativity in unstructured settings.
- *S*ocial types are helpful and empathic. They like to work with people and/or are skilled with words. They enjoy working with persons to inform, enlighten, help, train, or cure.
- *E*nterprising types are ambitious and extroverted. They like to work with people to lead, manage, influence, or persuade.
- *C*onventional types are accurate and attentive to detail. They like to use their clerical, numerical, and accounting skills.[23]

Holland has discovered that if one's personality (as identified by his system) matches one's workplace, a person will be happier and more content, stay longer, and be more effective. It is good to know oneself in this manner. Reading through this list and picking favorite activities—or kinds of people I enjoy—gives me a quick intuitive view of my Holland personality type. There are vocational inventory tests that can help one identify it more precisely.

The other aspect of this petal is to recognize populations of people with whom I would like to work. Is it children, youth, adults, elderly folk? Are they people of particular economic strata or need? Are there people with unique problems or issues to whom I feel close? These need attention as well.

My favorite kinds of things. These are the things with which I like to work. Are there tools, materials, equipment that I enjoy utilizing?

My favorite outcomes. These outcomes are both immediate and long-range. I will want to know what immediate outcomes I would like as a result of my work. Perhaps I would like to help produce a product, or provide a service, or offer information. It is worthwhile to ask about long-term outcomes. What are the things

I would like to do within a lifetime? Are there dreams, hopes, aspirations that need to be said out loud?

Rewards. The final petal has to do with *rewards—salary, level of responsibility, and others.* Here is the opportunity to reflect on what salary to request to provide for needs and wants. (Depending on a number of factors, the importance of salary may vary a great deal from person to person.) It is also the place to ask myself about the level of responsibility and leadership I seek and am willing to assume. (These two factors, salary and responsibility, generally go hand in hand.) It may be a place to ask what other rewards one would like from work—recognition, thought stimulation, adventure, or opportunities to explore leisure pursuits.

The preceding paragraphs have given a brief overview of the questions to ask in order to determine the "what" and the "where" of a career search. To gain tools and methods to answer these questions, turn to the books of Richard Bolles that I have cited, preferably in the company of a gifted leader and other committed searchers.

HOW?

After gaining this important information about oneself, how does one find a place of employment that fits the person one has discovered oneself to be? How does one get hired there?

The answer is that one obtains equally important information about possible job opportunities. Some written resources may be useful; however, this information is obtained primarily through interviewing people who are in a position to help. Our group encouraged and supported each person's doing many interviews.

There are two stages to the process. The first stage is an information-gathering interview. At this point the person locates someone in a field of work that matches her or his self-information on the flower at several points. For information only, the person asks four questions: (1) How did you get into this work? (2) What do you like most about it? (3) What do you like the least about it? (4) Where else could I find people who do this kind of work or, possibly, similar work that engages these interests and characteristics?[24] Each person contacted may have one or two pieces of information that are valuable to the interviewer. By putting all these pieces together, one discovers what one would like to do and for whom.

Equipped with the knowledge and contacts gained by informational interviewing, the job hunter moves on to the second stage. This is to go to the persons who have authority to hire people. Explain to those persons what attracts you to their organization and this work. Explain further what unique gifts and problem-solving skills you have to offer.

The job hunter will likely need to do dozens of information interviews, followed by hundreds of phone calls to obtain some job interviews. Tom Jackson estimates that a person will need to invest 200 to 500 hours of intensive effort in a job-hunting campaign. This will include 100 hours of job market research and networking, 225 telephone calls, 150 letters and resumes, at least 15 job interviews that may lead to as many as 3 job offers. One will need to make 10 to 15 phone calls to get one in-person interview. He points out that this initiative is so important because, on any given day, 80 percent of the available jobs are not advertised! He concludes, "A really good job hunt goes something like: No, No, No, No, No, No, No, No, No, No, No, *Yes!*"[25]

For those who find themselves discouraged by the rejections along the way, Strasser and Sena comment,

> It might be worth noting that James Joyce had difficulty finding a publisher for *Ulysses;* that the Beatles were denied a recording contract by a major record company executive who said, "We don't like their sound. Guitar groups are on their way out"; and that Clint Eastwood was told by one movie executive that, "Your Adam's apple sticks out too far, and you talk too slow."[26]

THE REST OF THE STORY

What was the job hunting experience of the persons in the group that I have been describing to you? What were the jobs and opportunities they found?

- The early childhood specialist is an independent consultant, evaluator, and tutor working with schools and psychologists. She is also an adjunct professor and educational tour leader.
- The middle manager in insurance found a position as a marketing manager with an independent insurance agency, offering specialized products and services while keeping in touch with changes in opportunities in his broader field.
- The displaced teacher spent a couple years doing substitute teaching as a way to provide income. Then she and her husband welcomed their first child. Two years later a second child was born. Now a full-time homemaker and mother, she reflects, "For the first time since kindergarten I am not in school this year. I don't know what the future holds, but this is what calls me now."
- The person with the new master's degree in library science found a position as a technical services librarian for a national insurance company.
- The mental health nurse is using her writing gifts to create resources for nursing education. She is also studying to become a parish nurse—to bring holistic health strategies to congregations.
- The cardiac-care nurse stayed where she was but made substantial changes. Aware that these nurses were "burning out" at an alarming rate, her employers brought in additional help. A disruptive employee was let go. Team cooperation and morale were built up. The nurse found it helpful to talk over her issues and no longer felt alone with them. This in turn brought an inner change. She felt more ready to prioritize what was most essential in times of high tension and to live with the unpredictable variations in cardiac care. She found renewal within her career.
- The person who was in clinical pastoral education is now a bivocational minister. He serves a small inner-city church and works at a factory making binders. His unifying theme in all this is making connections in a healthy way—connecting people to faith, children to adults, and the materials that provide good strong notebooks.

- The market researcher took an early retirement to pursue a master's degree in counseling psychology. He is now in his internship at a center that brings the healing gifts of psychology and religion together. While there are further steps before him, he feels the wisdom of the steps he has taken—from a research and engineering orientation to a people and spirituality orientation. He is finding that place where his "deep gladness" and the "world's hungers" meet.

I could tell much more about how each of these persons seeks meaning in life through a combination of employment, family and other relationships, spiritual searching, service, and leisure. They are wonderful examples of Builder, Synthesizer, and Reinventor career styles of which Carole Hyatt spoke earlier in this chapter. It is a privilege to share in their midlife career journey.

Retirement

We turn to one more topic in the area of life planning—retirement. It is a topic that deserves thought and planning by adults in the middle third of life. By age sixty, the first of us will already have entered this chapter of living.

Three considerations may guide us. The first is Richard Bolles's concept expressed in his book title *The Three Boxes of Life and How to Get Out of Them*.[27] Bolles suggests that there are three areas of life: education, work, and leisure. He suggests that at present, most people find one aspect of these overemphasized at each stage of life. When we are young, we have an orgy of education. As adults, we have an orgy of work. In retirement, we have an orgy of leisure. Life, he says, should be more than three orgies! As a first step in retirement planning, one might ask the related questions: How do I feel about the balance between education, work, and leisure in my life right now? Are there changes I would like to make? What balance of these elements would I like in my retirement years?

A second related consideration, as psychiatrist Viktor Frankl has written, is our most basic drive: the drive for meaning. He has observed that one can locate this meaning in at least three value areas: (1) creative values—what one gives to the world through one's work and creations; (2) experiential values—what one receives from the world in such areas as truth, beauty, love, relationships; (3) attitudinal values—the stand a person takes when faced with crises such as suffering, injustice, or death. Frankl's counsel is not to invest all of life's meaning in any one value area, but to seek as many aspects of these values as possible.[28] Closely related to this perspective is Strasser and Sena's suggestion that retired people have three basic needs: purpose, people, and joy.[29]

A third consideration is the unnaturalness of the "retirement at age sixty-five" concept. The first to set sixty-five as the age for retirement, with pensions and paid retirement benefits for persons beyond that age, was Chancellor Otto von Bismarck of Germany in 1883. Bismarck and his experts felt this was a supportable age, since few people lived beyond that time! Over the next fifty years, the retirement age of sixty-five was adopted by several private pension plans in the United States, and ultimately by the Social Security system.[30] Sixty-five as the age for retirement has become set in people's thinking. This thinking prevails in spite of the increased life expectancy, vigor, and ability of people well past that age. Jack Falvey states the issue sharply:

> I can think of few more damaging quantitative ideas than the age sixty-five (or thereabouts) retirement milestone.
>
> The age sixty-five arbitrary deadline has cut short many highly productive careers, and even lives. It has inflicted reduced living standards on people who deserve much more. It has caused involuntary geographic relocations that have separated family and friends by thousands of miles.
>
> In business, it has done grave things to retard growth, prevent risk at the expense of gain, and discourage innovative thinking in general.[31]

Even at that, for many, the retirement age is going *down*! Most Americans are leaving the workforce before they turn sixty-three. The U.S. Department of Labor estimates that by the year 2000, only one in four men and an even lower percentage of women aged sixty or over will be employed.[32]

In some manner, this thinking needs to be challenged. To that end, in 1987 the United States Congress eliminated the mandatory retirement age of seventy. Personal well-being, family financial resources, and societal economic resources will all be improved if creative and flexible thinking is brought to this topic.

How do people experience retirement? Many years ago, George Bernard Shaw suggested, "A perpetual holiday is a good working definition of hell." Ernest Hemingway agreed, calling retirement "the ugliest word in the English language." Pablo Casals, who gave virtuoso cello performances into his ninth decade, said, "To retire is the beginning of death."[33]

Surveys of contemporary retirees indicate agreement with these opinions. A Louis Harris survey reveals that 37 percent retired unwillingly because of a mandatory retirement age, health, or disability rule. Of those who retired willingly, 7 percent later regretted it. Nearly half of those who are retired say they don't particularly like it. Seventy percent of persons anticipating retirement hope to work after retirement.[34]

What does all this information indicate? It suggests that in actuality, retirement is a new career, deserving careful thought and planning just as much as any other career one has pursued. It may well have phases, with greater activity during one's "young-old" early retirement years, and gradually decreased activity later.

There is a financial aspect to this plan. A person will want to know that there are reasonable financial resources to see one through. This may well involve full or close to full employment for a few more years, for economic reasons, if not for other reasons as well.

There is a relational aspect to this plan. Married persons have reported a crisis when the pattern changes from being absent from each other 80 percent of the time to being with each other 80 percent of the time! This requires discussion and adjustment. Other relational hopes may exist—one might want to spend more time with grandchildren or children. Early retirees may still have aged parents who need care and attention.

There is an educational aspect to this plan. Reduced or free tuition at area colleges, elder hostels, and more are available to the older adult. These classes offer the chance to discover, explore, grow, and—possibly—retool for employment that has changed with the years.

There is a leisure aspect to this plan. While not the exclusive focus of retirement, attention to well-loved interests or the developing of new ones should be a part of one's life. We will speak more of leisure and play in a later chapter.

There is a work aspect to this plan. Perhaps one needs to discover that retirement is not necessarily an all-or-nothing affair. One may be able to negotiate phased retirement, or moving to part-time status. One may be able to maintain one's job, but cut back on the aspects that are too taxing, physically or psychologically. Perhaps one can retire but work as a consultant for one's company, or move to an alternative job within the company. Perhaps part-time work with another firm might be an option.[35] Samuel Ray has noted how older workers are redefining work:

- They are working part-time and spending more time on leisure pursuits and hobbies.
- They are self-employed consultants and subcontractors providing services to companies or even their former employers, but now they're naming their fees and hours.
- They are working full or part time at unpaid, volunteer positions to help create a better world.
- They are working as part of the new wave of executive and professional "temporaries," which allows them to structure work assignments around other interests.
- They are starting businesses in fields wholly unrelated to their "first" careers.
- They are turning former hobbies into lucrative sources of income.

- They are relocating to different parts of the country—even the world—and starting all over.
- They are returning to college and learning new skills and professions.[36]

The opportunities for personal growth and discovery exist throughout a lifetime, including the "retirement" years.

In Conclusion

In this chapter I have told stories and explored options and strategies for career journeys in the middle third of life. Very few of us will have a stable experience of one employment position for most or all of our career. Even those rare persons will need to adjust and learn. There will be changes and adaptations for all of us—new information, new career opportunities, new economic realities, jobs tomorrow that do not exist today.

In order to manage all this, we will need a spirit of openness and adventure as well as some basic skills to use each time the possibility of another change occurs. In this chapter, I have tried to provide some clues and guides for each of these needs. May your career discovery be as venturesome as that of the group whose experience I reported.

For Personal or Group Reflection and Discussion

1. Compare notes—how many jobs has each of you had since age eighteen? What was the longest duration of these jobs? The shortest duration? The average time spent with each?

2. How many careers have you had thus far? Are you dreaming, thinking about, or considering others? If so, what are they? Have you made steps in those directions?

3. Have you ever been fired? Out of work? How did your experience compare with what the chapter described? What were your most important resources for making it through that time?

4. How does your Christian faith impact your choice of employment and the ways you do your work?

5. You may want to invite successfully retired people to your group to talk about retirement planning and living.

6. Sketch out your ideal retirement plan. Parts of it may be clear and parts unclear. State as much as you can. Recognize the aspects that need further thought and exploration.

Resources

Barry, Dave. *Dave Barry Turns 40*. New York: Fawcett Columbine, 1990.

Bolles, Richard Nelson. *The New Quick Job-Hunting Map*. Berkeley, Calif.: Ten Speed Press, 1991.

————. *The Three Boxes of Life and How to Get Out of Them*. Berkeley, Calif.: Ten Speed Press, 1978.

————. *What Color Is Your Parachute?* Berkeley, Calif.: Ten Speed Press, 1995.

Buechner, Frederick. *Wishful Thinking—A Theological ABC*. New York: Harper and Row, 1979.

Dana, Jo. *It's Never Too Late to Start Over*. Briarwood, N.Y.: Palomino Press, 1983.

Falvey, Jack. *What's Next? Career Strategies after 35*. Charlotte, Vt.: Williamson Publishing, 1987.

Frankl, Viktor. *The Will to Meaning*. New York: New American Library, 1969.

Gruber, May. *Sky Hooks and Track Shoes*. Andover, Mass.: Brick House Publishing, 1989.

Holland, John L. *Making Vocational Choice*. Englewood Cliffs, N.J.: Prentice-Hall, 1985.

Hyatt, Carole. *Shifting Gears*. New York: Simon and Schuster, 1990.

Jackson, Tom. *Not Just Another Job*. New York: Times Books (Random House), 1992.

Morgan, John S. *Getting a Job after 50*. Princeton, N.J.: Petrocelli Books, 1987.

Ray, Samuel N. *Job Hunting after 50*. New York: John Wiley and Sons, 1991.

Srebalus, David J. "Vocational Choice: John Holland's Theory." In *The Encyclopedia of Career Change and Work Issues*, edited by Lawrence K. Jones. Phoenix: Oryx Press, 1992.

Strasser, Stephen, and John Sena. *Transitions: Successful Strategies from Mid-Career to Retirement*. Hawthorne, N.J.: The Career Press, 1990.

4

Marriage

RECENTLY, A MIDLIFE WOMAN came in to talk with me in my counseling office. Let's call her June. Mostly, she wanted to visit about her marriage. Jim and June's early years had been marked by a struggle to deal with each other, but also a vigor, a playfulness, and many laughs. Then their two children arrived. Both parents wanted the children, but the larger responsibility for them fell on her, or so it seemed. Almost too gradually to notice, the load shifted more and more to her. He withdrew bit by bit. June responded by investing herself enthusiastically in their upbringing. As this happened, other changes, slight at first, occurred in their marriage. They seemed to be less in touch, more withdrawn from each other— personally, romantically, sexually. These early slight tendencies had broadened by now into long-term habits, seemingly impossible to break.

They had now been married twenty-two years, and the children would soon leave the home. June found herself feeling great unease over what the future of their married relationship might be.

She sighed. "I used to find so many things that were stimulating and helpful for our marriage," she told me. "Books, magazine articles, talk shows, all held lots of good insights. The longer we've been married, the less helpful these are. If anyone knows how to do long-term marriage well, I haven't found it. I wish I knew."

June's lament has a familiar ring for many midlifers. Human relations specialist Eda LeShan has suggested, "There is no doubt in my mind that the toughest challenge of the middle years has to do with love and marriage."[1]

Family therapist Sonya Rhodes notes, "At midlife, things catch up with us. It's as simple as that."[2] Further, this facing of delicate marriage issues is not likely something a couple can settle once and for all in mid-years. It will be a recurring issue, requiring constant work and frequent attention. For not only marriage, but midlife itself, has frequent times of vulnerability. It has been known for some time that men between forty and forty-five are vulnerable to such crises. It has been discovered that men in their mid- to late fifties have yet another peak of vulnerability. Nor are women immune at either point. There is some truth to the concept of the "seven-year itch." From time to time, for visible reasons or no apparent ones, either or both marriage partners may question the quality and direction of their relationship. Fortunate is the couple that is equipped with openness and readiness to negotiate those changes.

The Challenges

Let's take a look at the many issues a couple may face in these years. Because of the wide variety of midlife marriages, probably no item on this list applies to all. Read selectively to identify issues that might illuminate your marriage. Midlife marriage is a complex matter, and it presents many challenges—children issues, midlife issues, cracks in the institution of marriage, and possible high-risk patterns.

CHILDREN ISSUES

Adjusting to empty nest after both partners overinvested in parenting. For many couples, the arrival of a child changed the way they viewed themselves. They changed their endearing terms from "honey" or "sweetie" to "mom" and "dad." Partly out of choice and partly out of necessity, much of their energy was directed away from their private couple relationship to the work of rearing the children. They may have found themselves so absorbed in parenting that they lost touch with each other.

Bill Cosby tells of the first vacation that he and his wife, Camille, took away from their children. They set some ground rules so that this could be a truly romantic interlude: no mention of the children; no photographs or other mementos of cuteness could be taken along; no involvement with kids. As they sat down to an elegant dinner in a charming old inn on Long Island, they discovered how difficult their resolve was.

> In the dining room, we found a corner table, where I sat down and began desperately trying to think of things to talk about. So far I had two: the plight of the dollar and the plight of the whale. I would have to pace myself with them or my mouth would be re-tired before the soup.
>
> After a silence of no more than five or ten minutes, I tenderly placed my hand on Camille's and said, "Have I ever told you, my darling, that they should let the dollar float?"
>
> "How you *talk*, lover," she demurely replied.
>
> "And speaking of floating, this is a tough time to be a whale, don't you think?"
>
> She smiled helplessly, and then I said, "You look so young and lovely tonight."
>
> "You've said that already, but I don't mind. If my loveliness is the bottom of your barrel, you can go with it for a day or two."

They struggled through the dinner and went for a romantic walk along the beach under the stars.

> "Just think," I said. "At this very moment, under these very stars, a little Cosby is wetting the bed." And then I piteously cried, "Oh honey, I *tried*! You don't *know* how I tried!"
>
> "Don't hate yourself," she said. "I was just about to suggest that we gather some shells for them."[3]

And yet, there is life after children, in fact, more and more life after children. Jane Porcino has pointed out that the average age for a woman when the last child leaves is forty-seven. She has reasonable expectation of another thirty-seven years of life. Two-fifths of her life lies ahead of her, after children leave home![4] For many reasons, including increased life expectancy, couples need to relearn how to relate after the children leave.

A cartoon shows a wedding scene. As the mother of the bride sits in the front pew crying, her husband says to her, "What do you mean, I'm all you have left? I'm all you had to start with!"

In one of the case studies that Sonya Rhodes reports, she tells a midlife couple who had endured some real strain with a troubled young adult child, "Parenthood has been a long complicated detour for your marriage. I believe that you can pick up where you left off and become husband and wife again."[5] Indeed, for many couples it is possible. Most marriages either become better or worse after the last child leaves home. The departure of children presents a couple with a question mark and the need to rediscover each other.

Dealing with resentments from over-investment and under-investment in parenting. More serious and widespread is the aftereffect of an unequal partnership in parenting. To be sure, some couples may have bought into traditional roles: one spouse will be primarily the provider; the other spouse will be primarily the nurturer. If both partners felt OK about this pattern, there may not be great damage.

However, one partner in a marriage may have longed for parenthood, yearned for a child, wanted a baby beyond all else. The person may not even have realized how much the child was wanted. When the child(ren) arrived, this person might have been amazed at the power of the attraction.

On the other hand, one partner may have felt uncomfortable and awkward around the baby and thus made a lesser response to the child.

Thus a pattern may begin, where one marriage partner feels left out and jealous. The other is overinvested in the children, probably oblivious to the left-out spouse's reaction. (Quite frequently, later on, both partners can remember the other's contribution to this impasse, but not recognize their own.) In the most severe cases it can even be said that a person "divorces" a spouse and "marries" the children. This does not refer to physical sexual incest, but to close emotional bonding and sharing.

This scenario is a frequent contributor to midlife marriage tensions. Some therapists believe it is the most frequent cause of midlife marital disharmony.

Living with the tension of young adult offspring who do not "follow the script" as to when to leave and stay away. The "old" practical wisdom was that children left home as soon as possible, probably at ages eighteen to twenty-one. The further wisdom was, "It's hard to have them leave—and harder to have them come back." Usually the returns were for short durations, such as college or work vacations, or furloughs from armed services.

These days it is much more difficult to enter the independent domain and to stay there. Higher costs of living, housing and schooling, divorce, job loss and layoffs, financial reverses and bankruptcy all conspire to make young adults less independent. Offspring may stay home longer, and return for extended transitional times (perhaps with a spouse and possibly with children).

We will speak of this more in chapter 6. Here we simply note it as a contributor to marital stress. There are at least two circumstances when the return of offspring is particularly stressful: (1) when the couple has unresolved issues regarding over- or underinvestment in the children, and the arrival home of a young adult child wanting space and resources opens old wounds; (2) when the returning offspring belong to only one of a remarried couple, the nonparent partner may well feel even more left out, put upon, and invaded, adding to a feeling of great stress.

Reordering life around the "midlife baby." Some of us midlifers enter marriage relatively late in life. Many postpone parenting for a time for a variety of reasons. Some of us may feel we have decided against children at all and then, under the ticking of the "biological clock," decide to go ahead.

And so some midlifers in their late thirties or their forties are at the other end of the parenting dilemmas—that is, just beginning them. They will not be exempt from the reordering of their time, resources, and energy. Hopefully, they will have experience and wisdom to do it well. At the same time, they will need to be prepared to have some long established routines interrupted.

In this regard, Ross Goldstein notes:

> A recent study of older mothers found that, compared to younger mothers, they have less energy, and more physical complaints, need more sleep, and require more support from their spouses, friends, or hired help. On the other hand, older mothers are more comfortable with themselves, and the self knowledge and self-acceptance that often accompanies aging makes them more patient with their children. They are more relaxed, flexible, humorous, and understanding.
>
> Late parenthood makes sense for a lot of baby boomer men, too. Many have not felt sufficiently grown up to undertake the role of husband or father . . . They are, by now, established in their work, and their financial resources are greater than in younger days.[6]

We will give more attention to this topic in chapter 6 as well. For now, we simply note that some marriages in the middle years may have an additional adjustment—the midlife baby.

For one reason or several, couples who have had children will find issues that are centered on these offspring cropping up in their attempt to establish a strong midlife marriage.

MIDLIFE ISSUES

Being in midlife with midlife issues, and being married for enough years for life to become routine—these conditions also have an impact on marriages.

The impact on a marriage of one or both partners' midlife crisis. Barbara Fried has noted that one's capacity for intimacy depends on a firm sense of identity. In a midlife crisis, when a person's sense of identity wavers, a person's ability and willingness to sustain intimacy is reduced.[7] This truth is the legendary cause of many marital hazards and breakups.

People speak of the "Midlife Terrors"—the terrors of aging, becoming decrepit, of death and dying. To shut out these terrors, one might abandon every sign of aging, including an aging spouse and aging children. Rather, one takes up with much younger "peers" to preserve the illusion of remaining young. One might marry a youthful spouse for the same reason.

When one casts aside a good marriage, family, and other relationships in such a fashion, people speak of the "Midlife Crazies." That image may be more accurate than people realize. Sonya Rhodes notes:

> I have found that some men—about 10 percent of those interviewed—react so extremely to midlife terrors that they actually seem to undergo a *transient psychotic episode* that may last up to two or three years.[8]

The wisest counsel for the person undergoing such terrors or crazies—and for the spouse—is to give it patience and time. However, that is often hard counsel to receive, for awareness of the shortness of time may be what is panicking the person in the first place. Still, cautions against precipitous decisions and actions are needed to preserve what might be otherwise good marriages.

Subjecting one's marriage to midlife scrutiny and decision making. While midlife terrors or crazies mostly come from the gut, this item is largely a head exercise—though mind and heart are very much a part of both of them.

If middle age is a time of life review, it is to be expected that one's marriage will appear on the list of items to be evaluated. Do I wish to continue in this marriage? Are changes necessary for it to be a fitting relationship for the future?

Persons tend to ask these questions pessimistically, at least at first. Sonya Rhodes, out of the experience of treating over two hundred midlife couples and interviewing another hundred, offers some corrective perspectives.

She notes that it is a most worthwhile effort to see if a marriage of ten, twenty, or thirty years can be rebuilt. Further, she notes that contrary to what many people feel, the longer a couple has been married, the more reparable their marriage might be. Crises may look more dire than they actually are. Strengths on which the couple can draw may have been ignored or taken for granted.[9] In these conditions, it is important that midlife persons take a long look at their marriage, perhaps aided by a skilled marriage therapist.

Making the way through long-term, habitual, possibly "boring" relationships. Some of the midlife problems with marriages occur because more of us are living long enough to experience them! In the eighteenth century, a couple marrying in their early twenties had only a 57 percent chance of both partners surviving to their silver wedding anniversary. Now, at least 92 percent have a chance of both surviving for that long. The average expected life of a marriage from wedding to death has increased from less than twenty-five years to approximately fifty years. Further, a century ago, a couple would spend 54 percent of their married life raising young children, compared to 18 percent today.[10] Along with longer duration, marriages have less child-rearing time than ever before. An important issue in modern marriage, then, is "What do we do with the extra years, including many child-free years?"

Too often the answer seems to be, "Not much. We become habitual, predictable, boring." Robert Lee and Marjorie Casebier point out that the root word *bore* means "to make something empty." Years ago, Balzac warned, "Marriage must continually conquer the monster that devours, the monster of habit." Lee and Casebier warn, "Habit, routine, sameness, emptiness, disenchantment, the feeling of being taken for granted, a blah feeling, a lack of any sense of value—all these are variations on the same theme."[11]

Vital exchange of feelings, interests, even conflict can interrupt the boredom of routine and break the trap. Ross Goldstein suggests that the core issue for many couples in midlife is that of growth versus stagnation. Often, he suggests, the third party in a midlife marriage is one or both persons' evolving self. The partners hunger for personal growth without upsetting the marriage too much. People also desire new life for a relationship which may have seemed to quit growing.[12]

Bill Cosby speaks of long-term habits in his marriage and how he and his wife deal with them:

> In discussing his marriage, a journalist named Michael Grant has said, "We continue to adjust to each other, but don't mistake it for a solid marriage. There is no such thing. Marriage is more like an airplane than a rock."
>
> Well, *his* marriage may be like an airplane, but mine is the *Hindenburg*: floating grandly through the fog, full of hot air and music, ready to explode. I am certain that I have one of America's better marriages; and yet the challenge of keeping it successful never dims, for Camille and I may be blinded by love, but we have Braille for each other's flaws. [One of Camille's idiosyncrasies] would be her asking me every night for twenty-five years, right after I have kissed her and said how much I've missed her all day, "Did you lock up?"
>
> I do not require her to reply to my affection in Byronic couplets, but "Did you lock up?" closes the flue on the fire of romance. Were I then to try to rekindle the fire by saying, *Dear, I've locked you in my heart*, she might decide to have *me* locked up; and so, I simply say, "Yes, I did."
>
> "Did you really?"
>
> At this point in our little performance in the theater of the absurd, she will not say, *I don't believe you*; but a few minutes later, she will go downstairs and check all the locks. It is nothing personal: it is simply that women do not trust people of a foreign sex.[13]

Cosby adds a piece of wisdom about the habits of long-term marriage: Keep a sense of perspective and humor about them, and they will not become boring!

Experiencing and tolerating the midlife gender role switch. In our middle years, some men and women begin experiencing feelings and attitudes and displaying behaviors often associated with the other gender. As we noted in chapter 1, Levinson spoke of this as "adult individuation." In midlife we seek a greater balance in regard to a number of polarities.

Males may decide that the "rat race" of career is not worth it at a time when females are discovering the excitement of pursuing a career. Men may be becoming more passive as women become more assertive. Men may become more nurturant as women become less so. The male may become more relational and emotional at the same time the female is becoming more driving and unemotional. Men may be becoming less competitive at the time women are becoming more so.

In midlife, production of the male hormone testosterone decreases in men. At the same time estrogen production is declining in women. This accounts in part for the switch, but it seems much more sweeping than that.

This switch brings understandable turmoil to a marriage. A person may complain of how boring and predictable a marriage is, but one has to concede that such a marriage requires a minimum of effort. You know who you are, and who the spouse is. You also know what you can depend on each other for, what each person offers, and what each person needs. In the gender shift, all that changes. The partners may not know who they are themselves, or who the other is. A marriage that had at least felt secure now feels shaky indeed.

Hopefully, increased awareness has helped this process be better understood. Each partner needs to understand that not everything is changing. The core of a person remains. Still, each partner's roles are evolving, very possibly for the better. Each person in the marriage is growing toward wholeness. This may be an occasion for strengthening their bonds and renewing their marriage.[14]

CRACKS IN THE INSTITUTION OF MARRIAGE

Contending with pessimism about the longer-term marriage. William Bridges describes a midlife man who senses a "running down" of energy for his marriage and muses, "Maybe marriages have only so much shelf life—maybe they're only made to go 100,000 miles, maybe you're supposed to get a new one every fifteen years. Perhaps this was just the natural ending."[15]

Up to fairly recently some social commentators were advocating "serial monogamy," that is, changing marriage partners periodically as the realistic way to cope with all the changes impacting marriage. Erma Bombeck told of reading a book that pointed out the high divorce rate and the troubled state of most other marriages. She reflected, "[I]t made marriage sound as exciting as a yogurt orgy. After thirty years of marriage, I felt like a truss in a drugstore window—dependable, serviceable, and downright orthopedic."[16]

Out of her work with midlife couples, Sonya Rhodes does not agree with this pessimistic view of long-term marriage. She points out that there are many advantages for partners and their families in keeping that marriage alive. The question she is most frequently asked is, "How can a couple keep a long-term marriage alive?" Most assume that perhaps they can have consistency in such a relationship but not passion. Her response is that while not all couples can achieve a satisfying long-term relationship that includes both passion and consistency, many can.[17]

Contending with the wear and tear of the two-career marriage. In 1976, the number of two-income families in America surpassed the number with only one paycheck for the first time. The number of two-career marriages has grown even more since that time. It is estimated that today at least 62 percent of all marriages have two wage earners. Quite likely that percentage is higher for people in the middle years.

The nuances of such marriages may vary, depending on the reason why there is a second wage earner. It may be for personal fulfillment; or it may be because of economic necessity.

Either way, this vast investment of time and energy outside the home has significant impact on a marriage style. There are many issues with which to wrestle. How will the family work—food, clothes, cleaning, caring for children, yard work, repair and maintenance—be distributed and how will it be done? The need for friends and fun—where can the time be found for such "luxuries"? What about the need for spiritual renewal—how can that be built into a busy two-career time structure? Then there are issues of finances. What money is yours, mine, ours? With two wage earn-ers, how are decisions made about money? There may be changes in the ways decisions are made for a family with two persons com-ing from a power base of earned income. And if one person is of-fered an excellent promotion that requires a geographical move, what then?

Too little is known about working out an equitable system of power, authority, responsibility, and decision making in such mar-riages. More wisdom needs to be discovered and shared about the biggest issue of all for many such families—exhaustion and time management.

When persons with these demands on their lives hear about the sensitivities and need for extra time and personal investment in midlife marriages, they may despair. Most of their energy is taken up simply surviving! Balancing work demands, relationship needs, and outside interests is quite an effort.

PATTERNS THAT INCREASE THE RISK

Sonya Rhodes has discovered that, in addition to the issues de-scribed above, there are some midlife marriages that carry greater risk of not being able to survive and flourish than others. I will briefly report her observations. She puts these higher-risk mar-riages into three categories: high-risk female patterns, high-risk male patterns, and high-risk marital patterns.

Recognizing and dealing with high-risk female patterns. Dr. Rhodes speaks of the "phantom self." This is a self identity that may have been ap-propriate earlier in life, but is being shed in midlife, or needs to be. Such a change is related to the "gender reversal" we discussed ear-lier. Rhodes points out that when this process is resisted or avoided, the marriage is all the more vulnerable.

She points to three phantom selves to which women may cling and which will not contribute to a strong marriage:

1. *The Little Girl.* To some degree our society has trained women to be "little girls"—to expect to be cherished and cared for by men, and in exchange to look up to, honor, and build the self-esteem of men in

their lives. In midlife, "little girls" need to grow up, not only to fulfill themselves, but because the men are discovering their frailty and need. The woman who resists this transition misses important growth opportunities and contributes to the stagnation of her marriage. (Younger midlife women may experience this less.)

2. *The Enabler.* Women are trained to give care, to nurture, to encourage others. This caretaking, so valuable a quality, becomes negative if she always puts others' needs and problems ahead of her own. This becomes an acute issue in midlife when self-discovery, awareness, and development are very much a part of her life tasks.

3. *The Eternal Mother.* This person is so invested in parenting that she is unable or unwilling to shift her focus from parenting when the time comes that children need her less. This person may draw so close to one or more children that her spouse feels left out and the children feel smothered. Without a focus on children, she finds her energy for marriage depleted.

Recognizing and dealing with a high-risk male pattern. Dr. Rhodes notes just one counterproductive male pattern, *The Tough Guy.* This is the man who expects to compete and win, to rise to the top in his work, to have great sexual prowess. He tends to be rational, goal-oriented, a problem solver. He takes pride in being strong, firm, and in control.

In midlife, some or all of this self-image may well crumble. The man who ignores or resists this change may be deeply depressed. Alternatively, he may try to crowd out awareness by all sorts of out-of-character behavior. This is where the "midlife terrors" and the "midlife crazies" come on with a vengeance. The man who fails to face this tough guy phantom self may well destroy his marriage. Or his spouse may give up on him and do so.

Recognizing and dealing with high-risk marital patterns. Dr. Rhodes also points out three particular risk factors that too often occur in midlife marriages and that are counterproductive:

1. *The Deniers.* The couple may practice elaborate forms of mutual denial to avoid facing unpleasant realities. This denial may give rise to family myths, shared beliefs that support the denial. While it will be

upsetting, the partners need to honestly admit their problems and face marital issues before the marriage can improve and grow.

2. *The Stallers.* These couples fear confrontation, and so they may allow bad situations to worsen. They may be aware of the problems but prefer to attempt indirect solutions in place of "loving confrontation." Stallers are similar to deniers and need similar corrective behaviors in their marriages.

3. *The Resisters.* In these cases, one or both of the partners has developed firm, long-standing, rigid ways of relating, which may have lost their usefulness. Still, they seem unable to face the need, to make changes, to adjust to changing realities in self, partner, and marriage.

Any of these patterns is undoubtedly complicated by yet another frequent midlife issue, *The Affair.* Dr. Rhodes notes that this behavior may have different meanings in men and in women. For men, it is often either a sign that the marriage has gone stale, or it is in direct response to their midlife terrors (I want to stay young and virile!). Quite possibly a woman's affair may be transitional. That is, it may be an interlude leading her to feel more confident about the changes she desires within her marriage. While it is regrettable that both men and women cannot find less destructive ways to express their dissatisfaction, this need not be the end of the marriage. Persons should avoid hasty decisions after an affair has been discovered/admitted. A rebuilding process may be possible.[18]

Paths to Renewal

What response have we made to June, whom we met in the opening paragraphs of this chapter, who wondered about long-term marriages? We have identified many changes and complexities that make the difficulties of such marriages understandable. Hopefully, these insights help people be more forgiving of self and partner. We have also pointed to strengths that may come with the years—strengths that the couple may take for granted. But there is something more to be said—there are paths to marriage renewal. Let's explore some steps along that road.

RECOGNITION/AWARENESS

We begin with *recognition*—recognition of many things. We may have to admit out loud that at a time when our marriages are most vulnerable, we seem to have the least energy to invest in them. Someone wisely noted that midlife persons should give careful attention to their marriages even if they don't feel like it. When we are young we want each other. When we are old we need each other!

We must also recognize that keeping a marriage alive means working at it. A starry-eyed bride once wrote one of the advice columnists asking how she and her husband could stay in love forever. The columnist responded, "That's simple. You work like a dog at it." As the years of our marriage lengthen, we discover just how hard we do need to work to keep current with each other and carry our just (and agreed-upon) part of the responsibility.

We also need to be aware of what changes may be happening in ourselves and our spouse on the midlife journey. With this discovery comes another—such changes will inevitably impact anything as multidimensional and intimate as marriage.

We need to be conscious of what marriage issues we are facing as couples. The previous listing was offered to help a person recognize what might be the source of pain in his or her present relationship. We may need to shed individual or couple behaviors that might have been fitting at an earlier time in life. Yet, even as we recognize what may be troubling us, let us assign no blame. None of us change in perfect harmony with our aging or the demands life makes on us. We may need to be patient with ourselves and with each other. Further, each partner may well have contributed to an earlier pattern of behavior. Marriage therapists have a term for this: "collusion." These are "unspoken pacts, or 'deals' with each other in order to maintain certain habits or patterns of feeling, thinking, and acting."[19] These various agreements, conscious and unconscious, make up what therapists mean when they speak of a "marriage contract." An honest question that deserves shared examination is, "What is our marriage contract, and what would we like it to be?"

MARRY, DISMARRY, REMARRY

As this recognition occurs, the couple is ready for the next stage of a journey toward greater wholeness. This stage involves a three-step process that people have described variously. In his book *Transitions*, William Bridges speaks of the three steps as "Endings, The Neutral Zone, Making a Beginning."[20]

My long-term friends, Ron and Marjorie Erickson, speak of "Marrying, Dismarrying (that is, making changes in personal and couple priorities and needs); and Remarrying (that is, forming new agreements and promises with each other)." I admire them, for they have modeled this pattern time and again. They married as teenagers, and their married life has gone through myriad changes—two waves of childbearing and rearing; education and career development for each partner, more than once and not necessarily in sync with each other; personal and professional pain for one or the other; a growing feminist awareness for both of them; and more. Now in their early sixties, they have shared married life for more than forty years and are still alive with care for each other. They have managed all these changes in each other by following a basic pattern: marry, dismarry, remarry.

Sonya Rhodes suggests a variation in this theme as the way that marriages stay passionate and vital. She speaks of a cycle of *conflict, repair,* and *renewal.*

Conflict in a marriage occurs when one of the partners introduces a new element. This might be a new need, a wish to redefine self, a desire to change some of the ways they have lived life together. The usual responses to conflict are arguing and withdrawal. Withdrawal will leave the conflict in an impasse. To argue without seeking a rediscovered common ground may lead to a sense of being in a stalemate.

Repair, the healing phase, occurs when a couple manages to move beyond conflict. Rather than smoothing things over or denying the conflict, they attempt to understand it. Learning the sources of conflict, becoming more self-aware, developing more empathy for a partner are parts of this stage.

In *Renewal,* the couple reexamines and actually reworks their marriage contract, the parts of which they were aware as well as the unspoken parts of which they may hardly have been conscious. New information about self and other, renegotiated mutual expectations, new accommodations are all part of this final phase of the cycle.[21] Many midlife couples might benefit from a marriage enrichment or a marriage encounter retreat. Such experiences might provide opportunity to take stock, to explore needed changes, and to make good marriages better.[22]

Dr. Rhodes recognizes that not all midlife couples can achieve renewal in all its fullness. There are some that she describes as "marriages of *limitation*." Perhaps some aspects of their marriage are good but they seem unable to progress on other aspects. Perhaps only one spouse is interested in change. In such circumstances, repair—perhaps limited repair—may be possible, but not the full renewal of which she speaks. There are many who may choose to remain in such marriages. As good as possible but less than ideal marriage relationships can be worthwhile both for the couple and for extended family ties.

In the midst of exploring this conflict-repair-renewal cycle, other couples may learn that their marriage is "time limited" and they may do better to terminate it. Rhodes suggests that marriages that do not survive midlife turning points have at least one of these four themes:

(1) a lack of strong sense of commitment in either partner toward the other or toward making the marriage work; (2) an ongoing absence of sexual or emotional chemistry; (3) a lack of conflict-free areas that the partners share and enjoy together; (4) continued conflict that dissipates mutual liking and respect.[23]

However, no one should assume a hopeless situation before doing some exploring. Indeed, if both partners seek renewal, lovely growth and change may indeed beckon.

RECOVENANT

This leads us to one more step, a foundational step, on the journey of marriage renewal. Return to, and reaffirm your covenant with each other. Christians are a covenant-making people. We believe that God has entered into a covenant with us corporately and individually, and we are called to make a covenant with God. Because of God's prior covenant with us, we are able to covenant with each other.

Ideally, the marriage covenant was expressed in the vows two persons made to each other in their wedding day. Quite often, it must be admitted that persons were in such a haze of stress, fear, and confusion that they were only dimly aware of what they were saying and repeating. Still, they knew that these were formal promises that expressed what they had long ago felt in their hearts and said to each other. While the exact words may have varied, the basic covenant was, "I take you to be my lawfully wedded husband/wife, to have and to hold from this day forward: for better or for worse, for richer, for poorer, in sickness and in health, to love and to cherish until death do us part." As Warren Molton notes:

> Marriage as *covenant* is a relationship in which husband and wife commit themselves to each other, . . . promising faithfully to respond to each other's needs and gifts. The covenant says: *I want to do life with you*. It is a broad and deep commitment, a bond of pairing and joining. So long as both are sworn, the trust is inviolable.[24]

The contract is a different matter. It is less permanent and may (indeed, should) change from time to time. When changing the marriage contract, couples are called to reaffirm the unchanging marriage covenant.

At midlife we have the opportunity and need to change the course of our lives. One's marriage will need to be part of that change. The pain and trauma of midlife may become the positive turning points into a relationship that is more full and deep than ever it was before. May it be that many couples arrive at Roger Gould's description of the successfully renegotiated midlife marriage.

> The old conspiracies are abandoned. In their place is a relationship based on empathic acceptance of our authentic partner, who

is not a myth, not a god, not a mother, not a father, not a protector, not a censor. Instead there is just another human being with a full range of passions, rational ability, strengths and weaknesses, trying to figure out how to conduct a meaningful life with real friendship and companionship.[25]

For Personal, Couple, or Group Reflection and Discussion

Note: If thinking about or discussing these matters occasions pain, impasses, or hurtful arguments, then it would be best to find a marriage therapist to aid in your conversation.

1. Compare the first year of your life together with the present year. Which changes do you most appreciate? Which changes do you most regret?

2. Make a list of all the things you most appreciate about your spouse. Make a similar list of all the things you most appreciate about your life together. Tell your spouse about these.

3. What, if any, are the ways that you would like to effect changes in your life together?

4. As you went down the list of possible challenges to marriage in midlife, which seemed to fit your married life? What midlife changes do you discern in yourself? In your spouse?

5. What concrete steps would you like to take toward the repair and renewal of your marriage?

6. Recall the covenant you made with your spouse on your wedding day. Discuss what that covenant means to you today.

Resources

Barry, Dave. *Dave Barry Turns Forty*. New York: Fawcett Columbine, 1990.

Bombeck, Erma. *Aunt Erma's Cope Book*. New York: McGraw-Hill, 1979.

Bridges, William. *Transitions*. Reading, Mass.: Addison-Wesley, 1980.

Cosby, Bill. *Love and Marriage*. New York: Bantam Books, 1989, 1990.

Fried, Barbara. *The Middle-Age Crisis*. New York: Harper and Row, 1967.

Goldstein, Ross. *Fortysomething*. Los Angeles: Jeremy P. Tarcher, 1990.

Lee, Robert, and Marjorie Casebier. *The Spouse Gap*. Nashville: Abingdon Press, 1971.

LeShan, Eda. *The Wonderful Crisis of Middle Age*. New York: David McKay/Warner Books edition, 1973.

Molton, Warren Lane. *Friends, Partners, and Lovers*. Valley Forge, Pa.: Judson Press, 1995.

Olson, Richard P. *Midlife: A Time to Discover, A Time to Decide*. Valley Forge, Pa.: Judson Press, 1980.

Olson, Richard P., and Joe H. Leonard Jr. *Ministry with Families in Flux*. Louisville: Westminster John Knox Press, 1990.

Peterson, James A. *Married Love in the Middle Years*. New York: Association Press, 1968.

Porcino, Jane. *Growing Older, Getting Better*. New York: Continuum, 1983, 1991.

Rhodes, Sonya, with Susan Schneider. *Second Honeymoon: A Pioneering Guide for Reviving the Mid-life Marriage*. New York: William Morrow, 1992. [Strongly recommended for any couple or group of couples who would like to explore renewal in marriage.]

Tengboom, Mildred. *September Morning: A Practical Guide for the Middle Years*. Elgin, Ill.: The Brethren Press, 1985.

5

Singleness and Remarriage

A s we continue to explore the issues we face in the middle years, I must admit to an omission. While the topic of the previous chapter—marriage—is vitally important to many, there are also vast numbers of middle adults whom it does not touch. These are the persons who are no longer married or who never have been. In this chapter we will give attention to those persons and to those who initiate a new marriage after the termination of a previous one.

The single population has been growing steadily. It is estimated that in 1990, 48 percent of all adults were single and 52 percent were married. (Some forty years earlier, an estimated 3 percent of the adult population was single—things have changed!) Recently, the U.S. Census Bureau reported that there were 68,310,000 single adults age eighteen or over in America. Of these, 39.9 million (58 percent) have never married; 14.5 million (21 percent) are divorced; and 13.7 million (20 percent) are widowed.[1]

Part of this growth in single population comes from the gradually increasing age of first marriages, but not all of it. Nearly half of all women over the age of forty live alone. Not quite as high a percentage of men are single. From midlife on, females outnumber males, giving the males a wider freedom of choice in this regard. Single women between the ages of thirty and fifty-four outnumber the men by a ratio of 128 to 100. This ratio increases with every decade of age after that.[2]

This large, fast-growing, and changing population of single adults is too little understood. Midlife singleness is even less understood. Further, the growing number of singles challenges research on life stages and midlife itself. After surveying the adult development literature, including those we explored in chapter 1, Carolyn Koons and Michael Anthony conclude that all of these investigations were built on a married model—they assumed marriage, and possibly divorce. They concluded "that few studies have been conducted using empirically based research methods to examine the developmental issues of *single adults*."[3]

Entries Into and Varieties of Singleness

Clearly, the large number of singles do not comprise a homogeneous population. We will briefly examine entry points into singlehood. Then we will consider unique issues for this particular group. After that, we will go on and look at a few issues shared by all midlife singles.

SINGLENESS THROUGH THE DEATH OF A PARTNER

Many persons become single through the death of a spouse. Their early tasks will vary with the nature of the death—was it sudden or gradual? Expected or unexpected? From illness, accident, murder, or suicide? These responses will also vary with the nature of the relationship—was it loving or estranged? Dependent or independent? Amply supplied with meaningful memories, or full of regrets and bitterness?

With all the variations, there is an unavoidable period of grief. This can be done wisely and helpfully, or not. In chapter 8, we will speak of freedom to grieve. When mourning one's spouse, one enters into that universal grieving. However, there are unique aspects as well.

In grieving for a spouse, there is *shock*, a feeling of numbness and unreality. Hopefully this will be followed by *catharsis*, achieved by talking and acting out one's feelings, bringing to consciousness one's repressed ideas and feelings. This needs to be done until the compulsion to do so is considerably diminished. During the months and years following the death, there will likely be some periods of *depression*. This is normal, healthy, and to be expected. It can reflect an impact so severe, however, that some persons suffer health reverses or even consider suicide. Depression is often anger turned inward, and so there may well also be feelings of *guilt* and many expressions of "If only I had . . ."

A dynamic of all mourning is *preoccupation with the loss*. For some, this may be uniquely intense with the death of a spouse. The person may remain inwardly married to the deceased, and have difficulty moving beyond that terminated married identity. Some people may need special help at this point.

A sign of moving out of this stage may be some intense *anger*. This anger may be at the deceased, oneself, God, or other people. It is a healthy step on the road to recovery, and may be a help in resolving any leftover depression, even though it is difficult for those standing by the one who is grieving.

Finally, there is *recovery*. The spouse is granted a loving place in history, and the grieving becomes history. The person begins the growing process of finding life after grief.[4]

It should be added that the bereaved person may also need to make major financial adjustments during this time. Sources of income and the way it is managed may change. There may be less money for all of the needs one faces.

This is a painful, difficult process. It will probably take three to five years. "Bad grief" occurs when a person does not allow it to take its course and tries to rush through it. Perhaps one will even want to remarry before having finished grieving a dead spouse. Also, some people find it seemingly impossible to break the tie with a dead spouse and move on.

While this is thought of more as a late-life experience, it will come to some in the middle decades of life. Four percent of all widows are under age forty-five. There are an estimated 854,000 widows between ages of forty-five and fifty-five, and 2.1 million between fifty-five and sixty-four. The average age of widowhood is fifty-six.[5]

Widowed persons face the task of reconstructing their life when their assumptions and expectations have been permanently disrupted.

SINGLENESS THROUGH DIVORCE

According to the U.S. Census Bureau, in 1985 the number of divorced people (nearly 15 million) surpassed the number of widowed people (14 million).[6] Clearly, there would be many more midlife persons becoming single through divorce than through death.

One out of every six adult Americans is or has been divorced. For every hundred marriages contracted in America there are fifty divorces. Many reasons could be given for this growth in divorce. In our mobile society, the severing of ties with extended family networks certainly puts strains on families. Women's employability frees some from what would have been unfitting marriages. It has been noted there are fewer practical reasons for staying married than there used to be. There are fewer children, and fewer tasks that persons in the marriage-family unit perform for each other. There may be unrealistically high expectations for marriage and much disappointment when these high but vague ideals cannot be reached.

There may not be as much certainty about marriage as a life-long commitment. Yet, as a pastor who has done premarital and marriage counseling with hundreds of couples, I have never met a couple that did not think they were making a lifelong commitment. Nor have I ever met a couple whose decision to terminate the marriage was not filled with great anguish and regret.

Even though society does not condemn divorce as wholeheartedly as it once did, still every divorce carries with it pain and sorrow, and some disapproval. Dealing with that suffering is the first task for the divorced person.

One obvious dynamic will be the *pain*, which can be longer-lived than most people will realize. Accompanying this is *anger*. Widely experienced counselor and singles ministry leader John Landgraf writes, "I have yet to meet a divorcing or recently divorced single who is not an angry person. If we define divorce-related anger as the reactive emotional response of a person to felt rejection, this is readily understood. Rejection, or perceived rejection, accompanies divorce as a wake follows the path of a ship."[7] Yet another dynamic is a feeling of *crisis*. This is one's inner response to an emotionally hazardous event. Persons who are usually self-sufficient may find themselves with more upheaval than they can handle.

Clearly there is *grieving*. This differs from the grieving of the widowed. Widowed persons may tend to idealize the deceased, while divorced persons are more likely to be upset with their ex-spouses. Further, there is a finality about being widowed, whereas for the divorcing, the "corpse" is still walking around. Perhaps the ex-spouse is causing even more agony through noncooperation, litigation, or new romances.

As persons look back, many realize that in their newly divorced state there was an intense time of feeling sick at heart and sick in body—some have called it a "crazy" time.

Something many people experience soon after divorcing is increased *dependency*. Some of it may be based on reality—there are all sorts of new skills, tasks, responsibilities, and decisions to face for which one feels ill prepared. Other parts of it are based on an inner reality of feeling very needy for the presence, love, and support of many people.[8]

Women going through divorce often experience severe financial consequences. There will be financial adjustments for both men and women. What is affordable and how can one survive may well be major issues to face.

Jim Smoke has noted the following keys to divorce recovery: (1) finding and experiencing forgiveness; (2) letting go; (3) getting my ex-spouse in focus; (4) assuming responsibility for myself; (5) assuming responsibility for my children; (6) assuming responsibility for my future.[9]

The difficulty of singleness through divorce is compounded if there are children. Dealing with the children's sorrow and fears, finding ways to respond to all their needs and, quite probably, working out some sort of custody and visitation arrangement with an ex-spouse are some of the beginning tasks.

Clearly, entering singleness through divorce is a momentous task undertaken at a most vulnerable time. And yet it may be a necessary and helpful step to take. Jane Porcino suggests that divorce can bring a sense of freedom to both partners if they have been imprisoned in an unhappy marriage. Indeed, divorce may be the only way to salvage the second half of life and make it the joyous, creative time that it can be.[10]

SINGLENESS THROUGH SEPARATION

Some persons sever all or most ties with a spouse, but do not divorce. Separation has been called a "poor person's divorce" because it is more common among lower-income persons. There are a variety of reasons people might choose this option. A couple may discover they don't want to be together but have no intent of remarrying. Perhaps the finances of divorce, religious objections, or the resistance of one spouse keeps a person from obtaining a full divorce.

Separated persons may have all the issues of divorcing people, only more so! Separation may well be a time of ambivalence and turmoil. Either or both partners may be caught up in vacillating emotions about the marriage and whether divorce is a suitable solution. There may still be thoughts about trying to save the marriage. There may be pressures from friends or relatives—either way. The separated adult may be contending with feelings of guilt, rejection, anxiety, worries about finances, and more. There may be questions about the best decisions for children in the marriage.[11]

SINGLENESS THROUGH DELAY

Throughout our society, the average age for entering a first marriage has been rising. There are many young adults and early mid-adults who have more pressing priorities than marriage. Indeed, for some, these priorities must be managed before they feel ready for marriage. These might include career achievement, relative financial stability, getting to know oneself, having an opportunity to explore, perhaps travel.

Many people, even while delaying a serious consideration of marriage, assume that they will marry someday. Indeed, it is not uncommon for there to be first marriages of persons in their thirties or forties. They have added ten to twenty years of singleness to their lives before marriage.

For some, by the time they are seriously interested, there is diminished opportunity. This may happen to women more than to men. By default, they may find themselves single throughout their lifetime.

SINGLENESS THROUGH CHOICE

Whatever the previous circumstance, some persons are single because they consciously choose to be. This may be for any variety of reasons. It may be a religious motivation, either formally or informally. One's faith community may require celibacy to be ordained or to belong to certain orders. Or one may want to serve in isolated or high-risk areas and not want to put a spouse or family at risk.

Others may be so committed to a career or discipline that they recognize they are "married" to it. Still others may have discovered a community of persons to lend support in various ways and so prefer to pursue their personal growth in that setting.

Whatever the path, singleness should be affirmed by the communities to which they belong.

Common Issues for Midlife Singles

Whatever the entry point, there are a number of issues that all or most single people face. Let's consider each of the issues single people mention most frequently.

LIVING WITH LONELINESS

Surveys of single persons identify loneliness as the most dominant issue with which they live. As Linda put it, "I felt as though some-one had outlined me with a black grease pencil. I was aware of every inch of my body, every thought racing in my head. While I was listening to my breathing, I felt so out of touch with others, so isolated, so alone. I wanted someone to talk to, to pour it all out to, but I knew no one would care to listen. I felt as though I was on a desert island, and there was no Robinson Crusoe in sight."[12]

Eda LeShan tells of a reunion with an old friend who had been widowed a few years before. When they met they hugged, and the friend clung closely. Then she said, "You have no idea what human contact, *touching*, means to me now. I hunger for it every day, and the only people who hug me are my grandchildren." Another wid-owed friend wrote, "I have enough of everything except compan-ionship and it is unbearably lonely."[13]

This pain of loneliness may be particularly acute among the newly single. This loneliness may impact one's well-being. Studies among widowed persons reveal a much higher health risk, for both physical and mental health, in the first six months after the death of a spouse. Also, suicide rates were found to be higher in the first year after the death of a spouse.

However, it is not only the newly single that experience loneli-ness. It is an issue for many. Of course, it comes to all people, in-cluding married persons. Indeed, single persons may be in a position to do more to avoid loneliness than married ones, who may feel confined to their own household to solve their needs.

When people are asked about the times when loneliness is most acute, the answers vary. Some mention mealtimes, and oth-ers bedtimes. A lonely crisis may come late at night or in the mid-dle of the night. For others it comes with the calendar, on holidays, vacations, weekends, special events in one's life.

Robert Weiss has noted that the divorced or widowed experi-ence loneliness on at least two levels: the emotional loneliness oc-casioned by the absence of the spouse, and the social loneliness that may come with the collapse of a network of friends and associates who were part of one's married life. These friendships may or may not persist into singlehood.[14]

One's loneliness may be self-chosen out of pain and fear left over from previous relationships. Or it may be imposed because one may be without a social network. Either way, persons need to take several steps to deal with this central issue. First, become comfortable with yourself. Enjoy the freedoms of singleness. Learn to become your own best friend. Cultivate the hobbies, pastimes, and pursuits that interest you.

Second, discover a sense of friendship with your God. To be sure, when relationships have ruptured, one's God may seem to be far away as well. And yet one may never be more free to develop a devotional, meditative, and listening habits, to be still and know that God is God. There are two terms to describe being alone— the one, *loneliness*, of which we have been speaking, points to the pain. The other term, *solitude*, speaks of the promise, the glory. Discover what is good and enriching and powerful in your life with yourself and with your God.

Next, one will need to negotiate or renegotiate some friendships. Perhaps some old friends need to be let go. They may be tied too closely to one's previous married history. John Landgraf points out that friendships don't just happen, they must be vigorously pursued. Further, there need to be local friends, within one's telephone area. He urges identifying the most desirable potential friends and actively pursuing and proposing this relationship. There should be at least one same-gender friendship and one opposite-gender friendship. Romance and sex should be excluded from these relationships. What is sought here is not romance, but intimacy, mutual support, listening. That takes intentionality and hard work.

Another response to loneliness may be the finding of support groups. These may be conversation groups for singles, or they may be mutual interest groups pursuing the activities one loves.

Yet another approach may be to take intentional steps about dealing with one's most lonely moments. This may be finding a cooperative housing arrangement with some other folks. It may be finding or originating a group that spends major holidays together. It could be discovering vacation "buddies" or groups.

While loneliness cannot be entirely eliminated, it can be reduced in new and purposeful ways.

DEALING WITH FINANCES AS A SINGLE

While all single persons may face some financial problems, these may be particularly acute for divorced and widowed women. One study suggested that women experience a 73 percent decrease in income during the first year after a divorce. The same study notes that the man's income increases by 42 percent.[15] Other studies have indicated that though there is loss of income for the woman, it is not quite that severe. For widowed persons, study after study reveals the financial burden to be the second greatest issue, right after loneliness. About 40 percent of all widows live at or below the poverty level. Only one-fourth of all American widows live reasonably free of financial worries.

John Landgraf notes several reasons why good money management is a must for the single adult. For one thing, when one has less to spend and only oneself to rely on, any mistakes are relatively more expensive. Further, financial fright or ignorance can propel a person into an inappropriate marriage. It is much better to know that one can manage, and then to make marriage decisions on firmer reasons. Again, singles need to be savvy about tax matters, for the government exacts a large tax bite from unmarried persons. Further, singles may not be able to buy a home, and that has been a taxpayer's biggest tax break. And further still, singling itself can cost a good bit of money. One may want to live alone, or go back to school as part of one's adjustment, or seek counseling. Each of these decisions may carry considerable expense.

For all of these reasons and more, midlife singles may need to become particularly skillful in money management. Out of his listening to many single folk, John Landgraf offers the following guidelines: Earn as much money as possible. If current positions are low paying, do intentional career planning and development to move to a more advantageous position. Pay yourself first—or second. That is to say, have a regular savings plan. Beware of debt—the only two purchases for which one should go into substantial debt are a home and an automobile, and on limited income, one may need to be wary even on these. Consider living without an automobile. Spend as little as you can. Barter—exchange services that may help two persons escape costly expenses. Avoid taxes—to find the legitimate ways to reduce taxes, one may need financial counseling. Check your Social Security credits—send in that card to be sure your payments are being credited to your account. Maintain adequate insurance, particularly health insurance. Even a modest medical problem can wipe out all of one's savings and assets without insurance, and health issues do increase through middle age and beyond. Hire a financial adviser—a qualified one—especially if the matters of which we have been speaking trouble, but do not particularly interest, you.[16]

MANAGING THE DELICATE TASK OF SINGLE PARENTING

We will speak of midlife parenting in chapter 6. At this point we simply note some of the extra responsibilities that go along with parenting when one is single.

For one thing, single parents need to assume a wider range of tasks. Economic provision; household tasks of preparing food, providing clothing, cleaning; and personal contact, leadership, discipline, interactions with children—all these and more fall on one person. This in turn leads to yet another need—to develop excellent skills in time management for the myriad responsibilities.

For some single parents, the divorced ones, there may be issues about visits by or to another parent, and possibly of joint custody. All of these involve constant negotiation and arrangements with an ex-spouse from whom one attempted to sever ties.

Child care and supervision will be another issue. Most single parents work, and care for the children who are young enough to need constant attention is a first task. As children grow older, the need for adult presence and supervision in years when children may feel they don't need it is an equally sensitive issue.

For single parents, above all others, money matters are apt to be problematical. In the parents' middle years, children may well come into the teenage and young-adult years. Teenage tastes can be very expensive. College educations and other needs of fledgling young adults are even more so. Costs may be high and the money supply low.

Along with all this, the single parent needs to evolve a parenting style. With the absence of a supportive partner, some single parents sense a collapse of generations. One's children often seem more like one's peers and friends. This may work for a while, but it may be problematical when adult perspective and discipline is needed in young lives.

With this wealth of tasks and strain of resources, the wonder is that many single-parent families function very effectively.

DATING, DEVELOPING A SOCIAL LIFE, COMING TO TERMS WITH SEXUAL ISSUES

Midlife persons may choose to move beyond a circle of nonromantic friends. They may decide to explore the world of "dating" again, either for the enjoyment of it or to seek a new mate. This may feel like strange territory. It was left behind years before, and the world has changed considerably in the meantime.

How does one find possible dating partners? Is anyone available in one's current circle of friends and associates? Will friends make introductions? How about the single ministries of churches? Are there possibilities at work? And what about these ads and video dating services?

What protocol, what etiquette now applies in midlife dating? May women initiate dates? What about the finances—who pays? In the busy lives of midlife singles, can one be more open about timing, for example, late nights?

Fortunate is the person who has experienced friends to advise and coach. Broadly speaking, it is quite OK to balance one's own needs and preferences, assertively stated with kindness and consideration for the other.

Yet another dynamic is sexuality and sex. What expectations do others have? What does one want for oneself? Because there are a wide variety of behaviors in midlife dating, one should be clear about one's personal sex ethic. One may determine that one will be celibate while dating. Another possibility is that one will meet sexual needs through self-care, including masturbation. Still another choice is that sexual expression will match the level of commitment between two persons. A tragic and urgent fact of life in making such decisions is the existence of AIDS, which is the third leading cause of death for those age twenty-five to forty-four.[17] The key questions are these: What do I believe? How can I deal with this important part of my life and feel good when I look in the mirror?[18]

ATTAINING SELF-ACCEPTANCE AS A SINGLE AND OF THE SINGLE STYLE OF LIFE

When Carolyn Koons and Michael Anthony, in surveying several hundred Christian singles, asked, "What do you consider the greatest advantage of being single?" both men and women gave the same four answers. (The order varied slightly.) They said the advantages are: (1) mobility and freedom; (2) time for personal interests; (3) social life in general; (4) privacy.[19]

Those are important advantages. However, in John Landgraf's opinion they are but part of an even greater good, the healthy self-awareness of being single. He writes:

Singlehood is a state of existence, a way of being. It is a condition of encouraging, affirming and maintaining one's integrity as a self. It is being willing—and learning how—to become increasingly self-aware, self-preserving, self-affirming, self-fulfilling, and autonomous (self-governing). It is taking responsibility for one's own well-being (total health and wholeness). It is making decisions for one's own life.

Further, he points out,

- Singlehood can be a state of high-level wellness.
- One can be single and sexually whole.

- One can be well married to oneself.
- Once wholly single, a person is free to have a life mate—or not to have one.
- Singlehood is always lived within relationships.[20]

From these people's viewpoints, there are two states of living that are related but quite different. One is being unmarried—whether widowed, divorced, or never wed. One may have this status thrust upon one without wanting it. The other is being single. In their opinion, this should be actively sought, cultivated, developed. Then, whatever comes, one will both have more self-direction and more to offer.

DEVELOPING A THEOLOGY OF SINGLENESS

It must be admitted that for centuries our culture has assumed marriage and assigned singleness a second-class status. This was true of the biblical setting as well. Indeed, Jesus and Paul were born into a culture that considered marriage and childbearing as both an expectation and a blessing. In a time that did not have a clear concept of life after death, family and children were one's immortality. To be childless and single was to perish.[21]

In the new age that Jesus inaugurated and Paul heralded, there were new hopes, new possibilities, new reasons for living. Therefore one could make new decisions about marriage and singleness as well. Jesus and Paul (in all likelihood) were single. They modeled that singleness may be an appropriate way to live life and that marriage or singleness can be part of one's calling. Indeed for some persons in some settings, it may be a better way of life than marriage. (See Matthew 19 and I Corinthians 7.) Further, there were persons before them in the Old Testament who—for all or part of their lives—lived in faithfulness to God as singles. Ruth, Nehemiah, Jeremiah, and Elijah are among such people. We need to follow this leadership of people in the Bible.

Whatever the reason for being single, the church needs a theology of inclusiveness for single people. As Rodney Clapp has said, "One sure sign of a defective interpretation of Christian family is that it denigrates and dishonors singleness."[22]

The Bible affirms that each person is the image of God, without regard to marital status. True, the Bible does say it is not good for persons to be alone. However, this is not a blanket endorsement of marriage for everyone. It is instead an awareness that each of us lives in relationship to many other persons.

The Bible speaks of God's unconditional love for each person and of God's spiritual gifts to each person—as individual, as single. One may know God's wholeness and healing as a single. Indeed one may be uniquely used of God as a single. For all or part of a life, it may be a very special place to be.[23]

Remarriage as a Mid-Lifestyle

In a midlife remarriage, the couple will have a few issues that differ from those described in chapter 4. Father James Young writes:

> The seventeenth-century British historian Samuel Johnson once said that remarriage is always a triumph of hope over experience. I have a psychiatrist friend who says he would never recommend second marriage—it's just too complicated, too chancy, too open to further failure and pain.[24]

Such cautions are well known. Yet there are many remarriages. It is estimated that at least one-fourth of all adults have married at least twice by midlife.

Emily and John Visher, pioneers in resourcing the remarried family, note five structural characteristics in which the stepfamily differs from the first-marriage family: (1) practically all members of the new family have sustained the loss of a primary relationship; (2) where the remarriage was preceded by divorce, at least one biological parent probably lives outside the current family unit; (3) the relationship between the adult couple in the household is predated by the relationship of parents to biological children; (4) role definitions are weak; and (5) often the children in remarried households have membership in more than one household.[25] Those matters alone do indeed make bringing together a successful remarried family a complicated task.

Further, all the family members will have previous experience in one or more families. Out of these, they will have a wide range of opinions about virtually every detail of family life. Bedtimes, food, the TV, how to spend holidays, what to spend money on, and more all need to be worked out. None of these matters can be assumed. That consumes an enormous amount of energy!

There is more. While a man and a woman may have fallen in love and enter this marriage enthusiastically, not all will share these feelings. There may be varying degrees of acceptance or resistance among the children in the household. If some persons are actively resisting, they may show this in a number of ways. There may be discipline problems, rudeness, acting out, and attempts to sabotage the new marriage. Rejection of stepparents by children can have a negative impact on the feelings of two people for each other.

Indeed, children and money are seen as frequent problems in second marriages. Making every attempt to help children feel OK about the marriage is important. So is working out understandings about involvement, guidance, discipline of each other's children. In midlife marriages, these children may be youths or young adults who have very little chance for bonding with a new stepparent.

Honesty about finances, including responsibility for children's educations and prenuptial agreements, may be important early steps to a sound marriage.

Some of the midlife marriage issues mentioned in chapter 4 may well be a part of a new midlife remarriage. For example, there may be the impact of either or both persons' midlife crises. A new marriage might be part of a person's denial of aging, of one's "midlife crazies." In such cases a person marries someone much younger in a search for youthfulness and a denial of one's own aging. Of course, not all marriages of persons with age difference fall into this pathology, but if this *is* the case, both partners are in for some disappointments and bigger adjustments than they may anticipate at the time of the marriage.

Such a marriage might fall into one of the high-risk patterns of which Sandra Rhodes spoke. An older male marrying a younger female may feed her phantom self of "The Little Girl." While this may be enjoyable for both in courtship and early marriage, it is unlikely to stay that way.

So far, we have been speaking of some of the sober issues and problems that midlife remarriages might face. It should be added that they present special opportunities as well. There is a newness, a freshness, an excitement. The partners have not accumulated resentments toward each other, nor has boredom set in. Hopefully, the partners have become more mature with the years, more skilled in negotiations and conflict management. They now have a new relationship in which to develop and enjoy those skills. They have not yet fallen into those high-risk marital patterns of being "Deniers," "Stallers," or "Resisters." Instead, they have the opportunity to build a sound relationship by facing each day's issues, by keeping current with each other.

In a study of eighty remarried families with children in the home, researchers found three significant factors that contributed to the strength of these families. For one thing, there was a supportive environment provided by relatives, friends, and community. A second factor was adequate family income. Third, the family had obtained professional assistance after the remarriage to help everyone in the process of adjustment.[26]

In yet another study, this one of remarried couples in their sixties, sociologist Walter McKain found seventy-four out of a hundred to be successful. From this research, he asked what makes for strong and happy marriages in the second half of life? For this population, he noted a number of factors: the partners knew each other for years before the marriage (perhaps one was the widowed spouse of a family friend); good health; good personal adjustment on the part of each; agreement to set up a new home away from the former homes of the two persons; a pooling of financial resources and adequate income; and children and friends who approve of the marriage.[27]

I would identify two factors contributing to strong midlife remarriages in addition to those mentioned in the previous studies. For one thing, the person needs to have recovered from the grief

and entanglement of a previous relationship, whether divorced or
widowed. The person needs to become fully single, as defined
above. Then the person needs to bring all those single strengths to
a healthy, open relationship. While time alone will not heal the
wounds, it does take time. Over and over again, single persons and
counselors mention the need for a waiting period of three to five
years.

Also, persons need to commit strongly to the new marriage
and be ready to endure some years of adjustment, confusion, and
chaos. In my own research, my colleague and I heard the numbers
four or five years (of difficult adjustment to remarriage) over and
over again. It was some time in the fifth or sixth year of their remarriage that couples began to feel comfortable, less threatened
when there was conflict, more certain that they would make it.[28]

Midlife singleness—for at least a period of time—will be the
experience of the majority of midlifers. A substantial number will
choose remarriage. These are options that raise midlife issues all
their own. But with intentional and mutual support, remarried
midlifers can create a satisfying life.

For Personal, Couple, or Group Reflection and Discussion

If you are meeting as a group that includes single and remarried
persons, it might be good to have the single persons sit in an inner
circle and discuss the first part of this chapter and questions 1–4 as
others listen in. After a time, others might want to raise questions
with them. If there are remarried persons present, the process
might be repeated with the latter part of the chapter and questions
5–7.

1. By which route did you become an unmarried person? What
was helpful to you in that process? What was unhelpful?

2. Which of the issues mentioned in the chapter are the most
significant ones for you as a single person? Did the chapter omit
issues that are important for you? How do you deal with these?

3. Do you agree with John Landgraf's definition of "single-

ness"? If so, how single are you? Where do you see need for growth in this matter?

4. What do you wish that nonsingle people knew about the single life?

5. Of the issues mentioned in this chapter, which are/were the biggest challenges in your remarriage? Were there important issues for you that the chapter did not mention?

6. The chapter mentions several items that contribute to family strength in remarriage. Which of these (or what other ones) were most helpful in building strength in your family unit?

7. What do you wish people understood about remarried families?

Resources

Clapp, Rodney. *Families at the Crossroads*. Downers Grove, Ill.: Intervarsity Press, 1993.

Deitz, Susan, with Anne Cassidy. *Single File: How to Live Happily Forever After With or Without Prince Charming*. New York: St. Martin's Press, 1989.

Kaslow, Florence W., and Lita Linzer Schwartz. *The Dynamics of Divorce: A Life Cycle Perspective*. New York: Brunner/Mazel Publishers, 1987.

Koons, Carolyn A., and Michael J. Anthony. *Single Adult Passages: Uncharted Territories*. Grand Rapids, Mich.: Baker Book House, 1991.

Landgraf, John R. *Singling: A New Way to Live the Single Life*. Louisville: Westminster John Knox, 1990.

LeShan, Eda. *Oh, to Be 50 Again!* New York: Times Books, 1986.

Olson, Richard P., and Joe H. Leonard. *A New Day for Family Ministry*. Bethesda, Md.: Alban Institute, 1996.

Olson, Richard P., and Carole Della Pia-Terry. *Help for Remarried Couples and Families*. Valley Forge, Pa.: Judson Press, 1984.

Porcino, Jane. *Growing Older, Getting Better*. New York: Continuum, 1983, 1991.

Smoke, J. *Living Beyond Divorce—The Possibilities of Remarriage*. Eugene, Oreg.: Harvest House, 1984.

Source Book of Health Insurance Data. Washington, D.C.: Health Insurance Association of America, 1995.

Visher, Emily B., and John S. Visher. *Old Loyalties, New Ties: Therapeutic Strategies with Stepfamilies.* New York: Brunner/Mazel Publishers, 1988.

Young, James J. *Divorcing, Believing, Belonging.* New York: Paulist Press, 1984.

6

Being Parents

IN THE MIDDLE THIRD OF LIFE, persons will experience changing dynamics in two important relationships. Over these years, there will be developments and challenges in dealing with one's children. There will also be significant changes in relating to one's own parents.

In this chapter we will explore some issues that concern being caring parents to our children. In the next chapter, we will turn to the concerns of being caring children to our parents. In the light of all the diversity, it is difficult to discuss mid-adult parenting in a few pages. The ability to bear children extends over a period of at least twenty-five years. As we noted in chapter one, the ability and decision to delay parenting creates wide variations in how people experience the life stages.

I shall focus on just two parenting issues of interest to middle adults in the 1990s. One may be of more interest to the younger mid-adults, the other to the later mid-adults. I will speak of the decision of many to delay childbirth until later in life. Then I will explore the experience of being parents to adolescents and young adults.

Delaying Parenting to the Mid-Thirties or Beyond

Growing numbers of women are delaying childbearing to their mid-thirties and beyond. In 1990, one in every thirteen babies was born to a woman thirty-five years of age or older. One in six babies was born with a father at least thirty-five.[1] This represents a substantial increase over the last decades. It is further expected that this trend will continue and births to parents over thirty-five will increase substantially.

There is an old-new quality to this phenomenon. Bearing children in this stage of life is nothing new. Over history parents continued to have children from their teens or twenties to menopause or death. It was only in the 1950s, 1960s, and 1970s that older parents were something of a rarity. What is different is that formerly, the child born to parents in their late thirties or beyond was the last-born of several children. Today, more likely the child is a firstborn. True, there have been other eras when childbearing was delayed. During the depression years of the 1930s, there were just as many firstborn or only children born to older parents as there are today. This was determined by economic necessity. Today, the decision is more a matter of choice.

Other nations have an even larger percentage of children born to parents over thirty-five. Four nations with widely varied cultures have a ratio of one in eight children born to a mother over thirty-five: Spain, Israel, Sweden, and Bangladesh.

U.S. Census Bureau demographer Arthur J. Norton, speaking of the 1980s and 1990s, noted, "The most important social change regarding parenthood is timing." The Population Reference Bureau, a private research organization, points out, "Delayed childbearing has indeed become the U.S. fertility phenomenon."[2]

In his book *Latecomers*, Andrew L. Yarrow explores late parenting, primarily from the children's experience. He first looks at this phenomenon from a historical perspective and from surveying adults who were children of older parents. He then draws comparisons to today's generation of older parents.

Yarrow notes that there are wide variations in the experiences of those who were such children. Some were the last born, perhaps into a family that had more than enough mouths to feed. Such persons might be labeled "accidents" and caused to feel guilty for the additional strain they brought to the family. Others were long-awaited and much desired firstborn or only children. Still others were the "ours" baby of a couple who had remarried after having families earlier and divorcing or being widowed. With all these variations, Yarrow points out that the people he surveyed identified certain advantages in such families as well as a few disadvantages.

The advantages include the following: (1) They were born to emotionally mature parents. Personal growth and readiness for parenting marked many of these parents. (2) They remembered calm, patient, and tolerant parents. These parents were often on a more even emotional keel than their counterparts in their twenties. When parents are more relaxed, there may be less conflict and anxiety in the child. (3) They were born into more stable families. Both marriages and careers may be more settled, giving the child a greater sense of calmness and belonging. (4) They recalled their parents' professional and economic security. Some of those interviewed appreciatively recall that their parents were comfortable in their careers and had the resources to provide for the child's needs. (5) Many were aware of being a wanted child with proud parents. One woman summarized much of this in her experience:

> There are many ways in which being the child of older parents is an enriching experience, perhaps giving you added maturity and sensitivity. I did very well in school, as I had been trained in reading and other "quiet" activities by my older parents, who weren't up to wild physical games and chases. I developed self-confidence from being taken seriously by adults I admired.[3]

There were also several disadvantages: (1) There has been a societal and cultural suspicion about older parents. Those critical of late parenthood have included members of the medical profession. A 1912 medical text said that later-life childbearing is "dreaded both by patient and physician." A 1950s text suggested that the expectant mother in her late thirties would stir a "feeling of dread and foreboding in the careful obstetrician."[4] Adults who were children of late-life parents recall feeling strange and embarrassed about parents' gray hair, wrinkles, and inability to enter into youthful activities. (2) Some recall missing activities shared by children with younger parents. Playing active games, going on picnics, having a parent as coach of a childhood team were some of the losses those children regretted. (3) Some sensed that the age difference made the generation gap even larger when they were attempting to negotiate value and taste differences as an adolescent and young adult. (4) Some felt they "grew up too fast"—spending more time with older adults. They felt they missed some of their childhood. They recall always being more comfortable around older adults than around their own peers. (5) Some recall a childhood filled with fear. This fear was for the health and possible death of parents or other significant adults. Being born to older parents may have meant that grandparents were already dead or died when they were quite young. These folks recall there being a lot of death in their childhood. (This was my experience. My father was in his late forties when I was born. He died when I was ten.) (6) This may have meant that children of older parents were cast into being caretakers for their parents at an early age. As teenagers or young adults, they may have had heavy responsibilities for parents or other aged adults. Or they may have grown up in a single-parent family, as I did.[5]

Against this backdrop of information from present-day adults who were children of older parents, Yarrow looks at the new generation of mothers and fathers over thirty-five.

He discovers a number of matters that have changed. For one thing, there are growing numbers of such parents. Parents and children do not need to feel as strange or isolated. There is evidence that late parenting is much more widely accepted. Then too, the older parents may well be more youthful, both in appearance and in the ability to engage in athletic play with their children. Improved health care for these parents may mean less health risk for many years after their baby's birth, and less anxiety about such things for the child.

Still, some deep issues face the late parents. Yarrow notes:

> The transition to parenthood is always a rite of passage that involves profound psychological and practical adjustments. For

older couples who may have more established routines of work, leisure, and social life, the introduction of a small, crying infant may bring unexpectedly traumatic changes to aspects of their lives ranging from sex and sleep to finances and freedom.[6]

There may be changes in self-image, and an awakening to other claims on oneself beside career. And there is a personal and financial commitment that will exist for at least twenty-five or thirty years. The child will need to be educated and provided with emotional and possibly financial support through early career explorations. Another question for persons who elect parenting at a later time is this: Will this be an only child? Being an only child also has advantages and disadvantages. Is that what we desire for the child's welfare?

There also remain some medical issues for those who choose to delay childbirth to the mid-thirties or beyond. It is known that infertility tends to increase with age. Further, there is a larger incidence of problem pregnancies. The involuntary pregnancy loss rate for women thirty-five to forty-four is twice that of the national average. Older mothers are much more likely to have cesarean deliveries at a somewhat higher risk.

Children of older mothers are somewhat more likely to have health problems. The most feared of these is Down's syndrome or other chromosomal defects. Nationwide, this occurs in one in every 800 births. It occurs in about one in 400 births for mothers at age thirty-five; one in 105 births for mothers at age forty; and one in 20 births to mothers at age 46. Prenatal screening is now available so that parents can know of this risk and make decisions accordingly.[7]

What is to be concluded about late parenthood? One possible conclusion is that choosing to have a child at the "early end of late parenthood" may have many of the benefits and few of the disadvantages. Intentionality about children is extremely wise. However, it is not always that simple! Readiness for the child is a complex matter. Finding the right partner, establishing a stable relationship, having a reasonable economic plan for supporting the child's needs—these do not occur in neat, easily planned sequences. Whether to be parents or not, and if so, when, deserves careful reflection and thought.

Parents choosing to have a child near the end of their childbearing years escape some issues of older parents of other generations. However, they face a wide variety of exciting issues all their own.

Being Parents to Adolescents and Early Adults

Up to now we have spoken of the decision whether or not to bear a child and of all the care and responsibility that decision entails. Now we turn abruptly to a subsequent issue: When that child is in teens, twenties, thirties, how do we relate to him or her? Release him or her? What is needed as a basis for that release? How do we prepare both the child and ourselves for it? What do we offer and how do we relate after that release?

This aspect of parenting has had scant attention. It is not known whether this deficiency exists because authorities have thought we let our young adult children go freely and instinctively, or because they did not know what to say! We shall try to draw together some wisdom and experience on this topic.

ADOLESCENCE AND YOUNG ADULTHOOD

The dictionary defines adolescence as that period of life in which a child changes into an adult. An adolescent, then, is a person who is no longer a child, but not fully an adult. In the history of humankind, this is a relatively new phenomenon. Up until a century or so ago, people moved directly from childhood into adulthood, or at least into the adult workforce.

Recently, the adolescent years have been given considerable attention. Barbara and Philip Newman have summarized those studies. They have noted that the early adolescent (approximately age twelve to seventeen) has at least four basic "developmental tasks." One is to achieve and deal with one's physical maturing. The onset of physical growth and maturity varies tremendously in early adolescents. With one's changing body, one begins to move into a more adult self-image. Another is the maturing of thought and reasoning. This includes increasing ability to develop logical principles and apply them to thought processes and decisions. It includes being able to manipulate more than two categories of variables at the same time. One is able to anticipate consequences of one's actions. Broader adult thinking begins. Still another task is achieving membership in a peer group. And yet another is forming satisfying relationships with persons of the opposite sex. In these initial steps from childhood to adulthood, early adolescents will spend more time away from their homes, looking to their group rather than parents for companionship, fun, intimacy, support, and understanding. The central issue in early adolescence is group identity versus group isolation.[8]

The later adolescent (aged eighteen to twenty-two) has further developmental tasks and issues. One task is achieving autonomy from one's parents. This involves the right and ability to make one's own decisions. It likely involves independent living as well.

Another task is the continued development of an internalized set of moral values and the testing of those values in living. Still another is that of career choice, at least reasonable first steps toward career choice.

The central issue is achieving personal identity while living with many issues that could confuse one. The late adolescent wrestles with questions such as these: What about me is most important to myself? To people who are important to me? What do I claim from my family identity and what do I reject? What is my society and culture expecting of me, and how do I respond? What do I believe and how do I want to express and support these beliefs? How do I pull all the pieces of me—family member, student, citizen, worker, believer, friend, sexual being, etc.—together into one integrated person? Such is the complex responsibility of the late adolescent.[9]

One of the recent developments in this regard—to add to parental confusion—is that adolescence is expanding. It is extending both ways. It starts earlier and lasts longer. Parents may see children aspiring to adolescence—in dress, makeup, peer group membership, interest in relationships with the opposite sex—at a much earlier age. Then, too, parents and adolescent children may have a long wait before the autonomy to which they both aspire is complete.

Quentin and Emmy Lou Schenk have spoken of persons in their late teens and twenties as NQA's—"not quite adolescents," and "not quite adults."[10] This is a time to work out that independence/autonomy in three major categories: financial, social, and emotional. This working out may take longer than either parent or child anticipates. We will speak more of this shortly.

As we noted in chapter 1, Daniel Levinson sees years seventeen to twenty-two as a "zone of overlap" when one leaves one major chapter of one's life (childhood and adolescence) and transitions into another chapter (early adulthood). These transitional periods are not brief, simple adjustments. Rather, during such a time the whole fabric of one's life is changing. These are difficult, scary, but exciting years.

In one's twenties, one has two basic but opposite tasks. On the one hand, one needs to *explore* all the possibilities of adult living— reach out, experiment, discover, enjoy. At the same time one needs to *settle down* and create a stable life, become responsible, make something of oneself, perhaps marry and start a family. These tasks may collide! One may feel one has made flawed decisions. Near age thirty a person may want to reconsider and redirect the choices made up to that point.[11]

THE PARENTS' ROLE

With all these huge tasks and fast developments in our children what role are we parents to fill? That is a delicate question! Zenith Henkin Gross speaks of the parent-child relationship at this point as the "orbital" stage "because it follows the children's launching into the world outside of the shelter of the home." It is a stage that, for a variety of historical and sociological reasons, did not exist in preceding generations, at least to the same degree it is now a reality.[12] We can best explore the parents' part in this by looking at a series of interrelated tasks, responsibilities, and issues.

Respect-encourage-participate in the young adult's search for autonomy. We are the parents who have been encouraging and supporting healthy independence in their child throughout the childhood and youth years. Allowing the child/youth to make as many decisions as possible is a first step. Encouraging self-direction in the use of money, allowances, gifts, and earnings is another. Still another is developing the skills for living. For example one needs to be able to select and care for clothes. There is also buying and preparing food and cleaning up afterwards. Then there is driving a car and doing basic tasks to care for it . . . budgeting money . . . working on values decisions . . . budgeting time and effort spent on schoolwork . . . making decisions about electives in middle and high school. All of these may be preparatory stages for young adults working on autonomy.

This transition toward autonomy may feel uncomfortable both to the parent and the young adult child. As much as possible, the parent needs to be encouraging and supportive of this step. It is the young adult's life, lifestyle, immediate and long-range direction that is at stake. One mother recalls sharing the same advice with each of her three daughters at the beginning of their college years:

> I will never relinquish my right to give advice, but at this point you are no longer obliged to take it. I have done what I can to give you the equipment to make your own decisions. Never let anyone else tell you what to do. Never make a decision and say, "she made me do it." If you choose drugs, sleeping around, whatever, it will be your choice. Don't close any doors behind you. Don't do something because it's expedient.[13]

This search for autonomy is complicated because, especially in the early years, it is never quite complete. One student told me, "Most of the time I love being on my own. However, when I get sick, I want my mom!" Both parent and young adult may pop in and out of two styles of relating—parent-child or adult-adult. Early in young adulthood, there may be a few extraordinary times when parents would step in—a severe illness, an overwhelming depression, a person's being drawn into illegal activities. For the vast majority of the time, however, it is best to allow/support/encourage children to make their own decisions and to live with the consequences.

Yielding to this drive for autonomy might hurt. The young adult may reject parents' values, lifestyle, faith, and church. The child may insist that she or he will never enter a parent's occupation—even if that appears to be a good fit.

For many, the issue of independence/autonomy will be sharpest in the earlier years. If both sides negotiate it successfully, they may mellow on this topic. However, it will never entirely go away.

This snuck up on me in a gentle way one day. One of our daughters, fresh out of college and in her first job, came home for a visit. Glad that I had taken up jogging, she told me she wanted to buy me a pair of running shoes for a Father's Day/birthday present. I responded, "Honey, you can't afford an expensive gift like that." She snapped, "Don't you tell me what I can afford!" I picked out the shoes and let her pay.

Participate in and support the young adult's decisions and actions that help make the transition to adulthood. In these years, the adolescent/young adult will make life-affecting decisions and begin momentous tasks. In the late high-school years, the young person must choose a plan for after high school. Traditionally there have been three choices: employment; military service; and college or some other post-high-school training. The trend is toward a decreased availability of jobs for persons with a high-school education, at least jobs that pay more than minimum wage and that hold the promise of career development and advancement. Military service opportunities are also decreasing.

Evidence everywhere is that the fastest-growing occupations with the most open-ended futures are those that require educational preparation. Increasingly the high-school person's decision probably will be to attend college, technical school, or university. This brings one to another decision—which institution of higher education? This, too, is a complicated question! In the United States there are three thousand degree-granting institutions and another ten thousand that award various kinds of certificates. Selecting a school of the right size and fitting location with offerings that interest one—a school that will challenge the student and that is affordable—is a complex, several-stage process. I recall the excitement and strain of this decision with each of my children. One of my children wanted to see and consider as many of those three thousand institutions as possible!

Having made that choice, the next task is to survive and succeed in that setting. Coburn and Treeger give a picture of what that task is like for the person who elects a school away from home:

> You are leaving behind everyone you know and moving to a new place where you have made a commitment to spend the next four years of your life.
>
> When you arrive in this strange place, you look around and see a landscape of unfamiliar faces. A lot of these people talk differently from you; they have strange accents and use expressions you've never heard before. Some of them wear clothes that are different too. They all look smart, confident, and outgoing.
>
> No one here knows anything about the status you had in your previous position—or about any of your past accomplishments.
>
> You have left behind your family, friends, colleagues—all the people who are important in your life.
>
> You're not too sure where anything is or who might be able to help you.
>
> You have to share a small room with a perfect stranger. There are no set guidelines about bedtime, use of the phone, stereo, radio, or entertaining guests. You have to negotiate everything.
>
> You have more work to do than ever before, but you're not too sure how you will be evaluated or what people will want from you. You may not get your first evaluations for many weeks.
>
> You have a lot of unscheduled time and there are plenty of distractions: sports centers, concerts, movies, parties, clubs—and lots of attractive potential partners.
>
> You have to handle financial and housekeeping matters that used to be done for you or, at least, you shared.

You're not too sure where your work and new relationships are
heading and you don't know where or how you will ever fit into
this new place. But everyone has told you that your whole future
depends on your doing well during these four years—preferably
better than those other bright, confident people who live here
with you.[14]

Then, having negotiated all those adjustments, one will need
to find a specialization, choose a major to pursue and identify
some potential work and career applications of that interest.

The next task will be to discover an area of employment and
land a job. Then, as the person tries to succeed, he or she must
also ask, "Do I fit here—or at least will I fit when I gain access to
wider opportunities in this field?" Perhaps the answer will be no.
Then, perhaps, we need to hear Luther Otto's reassuring words:

We live in a forgiving society. People can change jobs. They need
not be stuck. They can always go back to school or get new training. True, the options foreclose as we get older, but we oldsters
need to remember that our young people still have time and they
still have options. They have an advantage. They can always start
over. Let them—indeed, help them—play out their options.[15]

All of these pressing responsibilities are concurrent with one
working out one's philosophy and style of life, possibly looking for
a loving companion, perhaps marrying that person, maybe starting a family.

While parents are aware of all these decisions and tasks, they
may feel confused and uncertain about what they can offer. After
all, is not the young adult who is doing this also seeking autonomy
and independence?

The best wisdom seems to be that parents are not shut out
from these important decisions. However, their role must adjust.
Luther Otto and associates have studied and interviewed thousands of young adults in the ten to fifteen years after high school.
Overwhelmingly, he received two responses from these young
adults: (1) they would like more help in discovering and adjusting

to a career; and (2) one of the sources from which they would like more help was their own parents. One young adult's comment is typical of many others: "Maybe this is passing the buck, but I think my parents left my future pretty much up to me. . . . A little more guidance of direction would have helped me to define a better future for myself."[16] As a mid-adult parent, my first response to that quote is defensive. It seems that we parents are considered wrong if we say too much or if we say too little. Then I need to move beyond my defensive response and ask some deeper questions.

For example, how much parental input is desired? When it is wanted? How it should be given? We know what we should *not* be—we should not be the authorities deciding for our children. We need to find a new way.

One model may be that the parent becomes a *consultant* to the young adult child. A consultant is called in when wanted. The consultant can give the best of his or her wisdom and expertise. At the same time a consultant knows that the "client" can accept or reject, use or refuse the perspective offered.

Yet another model may be that parent and young adult child become *partners* in this quest. Certainly both have a stake in the issues and decisions. The confusion arises as to who is the senior partner and who is the junior partner. When making these decisions it is one person's life, and (largely, at least) the other person's money that is involved. One partner is older, and for a number of years made all or most of the decisions. What is needed is a renegotiated partnership. The young adult becomes the prime or lead partner. The parent makes clear what financial involvement he or she can willingly offer, and what other perspectives, help, or wisdom he or she has available.

Still another model might be *assertive, openly communicating friends*. In this relationship, both learn to say openly what they want and need and what they don't want or need from the other. We will speak of this in more detail later in this chapter.

Certainly, this is a very personal and individual matter. It will vary from family to family, from child to child within the same family, and from month to month and year to year.

Somehow, in some way, parent and child need to develop the teamwork that violates no one and supports successful transitions from childhood to adulthood.

Negotiate money matters in a way that is caring and respectful and encourages growth. There will be several occasions when parents and young adult children will need to deal with each other about money. Let's look at those.

The first time may be in dealing with college expenses. When parents and child are filling out applications for student aid, they may have opportunity to be open and candid with each other about money. What resources does our family have and how much of a strain will it be to provide this education? This can be an important time, not only in calculating college costs but in being open and candid, parent to young adult child, about the family financial situation.

As applications for admission and financial aid are made, the family will encounter some realities and assumptions on the part of the institutions to which they apply. It is assumed that the family and student bear primary responsibility for meeting college education costs. Within the family's ability to pay, they are expected to do so. While there are some merit financial aid awards based on high grades or achievement in some area (usually sports), these are quite a small part of financial aid today. Most of it is awarded on a determination of family need.

Therefore the family will need to supply information about income, savings, assets, debts, liabilities, size of family, number of persons in college. (Much information is based on federal income-tax forms. These are the years you'll want to do those income-tax calculations early!) A formula is then applied to estimate what the family and student can pay toward the costs of attending a particular institution.

Any aid will be given according to a "package concept." The total aid may have three parts: (1) "gift aid"—scholarships and grants that do not have to be repaid; (2) loans that do have to be repaid; (3) work grants that involve obligation on the part of the student. The amount of aid in the form of loans is rapidly increasing. A student may well leave college with a debt of thousands of dollars. There needs to be advance discussion as to whether this debt is the responsibility of the student, of the family, or is shared in some way. Parents and child may also want to explore whether there are ways to keep this debt to a minimum. This is especially important if the young adult is going into a field that does not have high compensation.

There also needs to be discussion about what, if any, part of the college expense is the student's responsibility. Circumstances may have changed since parents were students. The number of persons who earn their way through school, or a substantial part of it, is shrinking. Most summer jobs and student employment during the year is at minimum wage. One estimate is that the student who works twelve hours a week (the national average) at the minimum wage can expect to earn 6 percent of an annual college bill.

The broad expenses—tuition, housing, food—can be accurately anticipated. There is much that will need mutual exploration. The costs of books, living expense, spending money will need to be worked out. Keeping an accurate record of what a student spends during the first couple of months at school will help determine a monthly allowance for such items.

Still another issue needs to be faced—are there expectations that go with this money? Are there actions that would cause the parents to choose not to invest it the next semester? Most parents will not want to put a guilt "after all we've done for you" trip on their children. On the other hand they may not want to communicate an "anything goes" attitude either. They are, after all, investing thousands of dollars. Do they expect that the student will want to be at college? Do they expect basic effort, evidenced by a reasonable grade point average? Perhaps yes, perhaps no. Parents may know their child well enough to feel such things need not be said. Whatever assumptions and expectations go with the financial support should be clearly communicated.

Still other money matters will come up. At college, one may come upon fascinating opportunities, each with additional cost. What about a year of study abroad? (One parent of limited means told her child that as parent she would provide the same amount she did every semester. The child would have to figure out how to make up the difference.) How about a spring break with friends on the slopes or beaches? What about leaving college for a year to travel with some international service, performing, or religious group? One of my daughters asked her mother and me to work with her to make possible a year with the traveling group "Up With People." She was responsible about wanting to do everything she could to earn the required money. Still it required a juggling of family finances to make it possible. If parents and college children speak to each other only about money, they will keep talking with each other!

Money matters will not end when your child achieves a baccalaureate degree or finishes tech school. For one thing, in many fields, a first degree is not enough. Young adults may feel the need to pursue graduate education and may turn to families for assistance.

Further, when education is finished, other needs and emergencies may arise. There may be crises that occasion financial need. A person may not be able to find a job or may be fired. Divorce may bring financial crisis with it. There may be injury or illness.

Then, too, children may ask parents to help out with needs or desires that are real, though not emergencies. There may be requests for help with a down payment on a house, up-front finances for starting a business, support while a young adult tries to gain access to a competitive field such as professional acting or music.

These topics come up frequently. A recent survey by the American Board of Family Practice revealed that 89 percent of middle adults reported assisting an adult child with financial needs. Zenith Henkin Gross, who surveyed five hundred mothers of young adult children, ranked money second among the topics that cause disagreement between parents and children. The first-ranked topic, lifestyle, and the third-ranked topic, lack of children's motivation, were closely related to money concerns as well.[17]

The following are among the shared discoveries of those who have handled money matters with adult children well:

1. Parents want to respond with help to real need *as the parents perceive it.* Loss of an apparently secure job, divorce, illness, accident are among the needs they would mention.

2. As to other requests for money, parents want the freedom to say yes or no and to do so without guilt. Parents will want to consider not only their own resources and willingness, they will want also to consider the best interest of the one making the request. From their perspective, the young adult child's best interest may be served by saying no.

3. Many money issues are about other than money and more than money. They may be about love, acceptance, reassurance, competition, jealousy, greed. Persons may need help in sorting out the money decision from the other emotional issues that are bound up in it.

4. When money changes hands, parents and children need to be quite clear whether this is a gift or a loan. If it is a loan, they are well advised to put it on a business basis. What interest, if any, will be charged? When should payments begin and when is final payment due? Most advise a simple, signed contract. Parents who do this say that, difficult as it is, it saves heartache later.

5. When parents receive a request, they need also to consider justice and fairness to the siblings of the one making the request. They will also need to arrive at their family's definition of justice—is it same-size gifts to each? Or is it equally compassionate response to each need—within the family's ability?

6. Married parents may not agree with each other as to what is a fitting response to a particular money request. They will do well not to let such decisions come between them. Perhaps, if they both have discretionary money, the parent who wishes to respond should do so. Perhaps they will need to compromise, both with each other and with the child making the request.[18]

In this manner, money decisions become occasions by which parents and young adults work out their changing relationship. (For a more detailed discussion of all these matters of relating to young adult children, see *Discoveries: Expanding Your Child's Vocational Horizons.*[19])

Respond in a productive way to young adult children who remain home and those who return home to live. Each of my wife's and my three children left home for college at about age eighteen. Parents and children both assumed that, while they might return for summer vacations and school holidays, they would not reside in our home beyond that. That expectation has proved true.

I have friends, midlife people, whose three children did not leave home at age eighteen. They stayed home, pursued part-time jobs and some schooling. Two left for an apartment for a time. However, the combination of the high expense and some scary things in the apartment complex caused them to return home. The parents weren't quite sure when the "launch" for each of their children would be. It appears that my friends' experience is increasingly widespread.

There are two things that are happening with growing frequency between parents and young adult children. First, young adult offspring are staying home longer. More than half of young adults age twenty to twenty-four are now living at home. This is a 50 percent increase from 1970.[20] Second, many young adults who left their families of origin find it necessary to return to their parents' home. Of the mothers that Zenith Henkin Gross surveyed, well over 10 percent had had young adult children return for a time. These stays varied in time from three months to two years or longer.

Many reasons may contribute to the delay in leaving home. Minimum-wage jobs may not pay enough for housing and other needs. Opportunities in military service, for generations the way some young adults have left home, are radically decreasing. The first years of schooling may be at a local college, due either to personal preference or family finances. Many young adults are marrying at an older age, and so they may not feel it is necessary to leave home as a single.

When young adults have left and return home, it is often because of some crisis or tragedy. There may be a job loss, and possibly bankruptcy. There may be a serious illness, injury, or addiction. It could be a divorce. Whatever the reason, there may be much pain that occasions the journey home.

Gross comments, "There seems little question that the weaning of America is taking a long time."[21] Okimoto and Stegall reflect:

> Where did so many of us get the idea that fully functioning adulthood occurs at age eighteen? In reality, adult children often try their wings, fall on their faces, and return home to regroup, recoup, and eventually try again. People, like flowers, bloom at different rates, and some young adults take longer to mature than others.[22]

Parents are apt to have two overwhelming feelings when an adult child returns home in crisis. On the one hand, there is the thought, "How did I fail as a parent if my child can't make it?" This is likely matched by some real crises in the young adult's feelings about self. There is also the thought, "How can we make this work, and what will it cost all of us to survive this?" The young adult may not be thinking about that question—after all, this is the home where one was a child and youth.

Therein lies a potential problem. Upon returning home, it may be all too easy for the young adult to regress to childhood or adolescent behavior. This may mean falling into a pattern of being cared for and provided for—no expenses, no concerns, while mom cooks, launders, irons, and generally takes care of the "child."

We can learn from those who experienced such returns as disasters and from those who felt good about them. There are some basic ingredients that will contribute to successful intergenerational living:

- Agree at the outset that this will be a reasonably short time span with defined limits.
- Negotiate ground rules for sharing the space and living arrangements. Persons' needs for privacy, what will be shared, and what is each person's own responsibility should be discussed.

- Discuss money. It should be agreed that as soon as possible, the young adult will make a financial contribution to household expenses, especially if the young adult has a job or obtains one.
- Parents should continue their own lifestyle as best they can in the new circumstances. If there are aspects of their offspring's behavior that they cannot tolerate (live-in partners or illegal drugs, for example), they should make that clear.
- Parents may want to introduce the possibility of the need for personal and/or family counseling. If the young adult is depressed, suicide-prone, mentally ill, having difficult post-divorce adjustments, or immature, professional help may be needed. A family therapist may be helpful if the family cannot work out the intergenerational living arrangements.[23]

These arrangements may make it possible for the parents to survive and for the young adult to feel like an adult in the parents' home. At the same time, the parents will need to recognize that this person returning to their home is an adult, with a right to adult decisions. Okimoto and Stegall suggest these as adult territories where personal decision should be respected:

1. *Food.* Adults have the right to eat what they like, when they want to.
2. *Sleep.* Adults have the right to sleep as much or as little as they like.
3. *Appearance* (clothing, hair, makeup, jewelry). Adults have the right to wear whatever clothing, makeup, or jewelry they choose.
4. *Friends.* Adults have the right to choose their friends.
5. *Lovers.* Adults have the right to choose their lovers.
6. *Jobs.* Adults have the right to choose their own job.
7. *Money.* Adults have the right to spend their money as they choose.[24]

The exception is if in exercising these rights, one directly affects the rights of others. A clear expectation of mutual respect for each other's rights must be asserted.

There are two sets of circumstances that may make this "survival plan" even more difficult. The first case is if the returning young adult is a stepchild to one of the parents. Two acquaintances or strangers, lacking bonding and relationship building, may need to enter a quite intimate experience, sharing one's space and living. The second case is when the young adult returns with a child or children. The parents/grandparents have even more issues—how not to meddle, but enter into the life of these children, without becoming unduly involved in raising them.

While the survival strategies I have described are important, there is a larger concern. Parents and young adults want to complete the unfinished business that caused them to be together again. Okimoto and Stegall responded to the question, "What do adult children need from us at this time?" They point out that parents need to start with these young adults where they are "confused, injured, disillusioned, embarrassed, floundering, ashamed."[25] They need their parents' empathy in their struggles. The young adult may also need a hopeful viewpoint from parents—that the parents consider this a temporary setback from which they will recover. There may also be a need to rekindle their confidence and competence by succeeding at something. As we have indicated, parents need to have respect for their young adult children's autonomy, especially in a time when they may not feel they deserve it. This respect for autonomy includes expectation of managing their own self-care tasks. They need acceptance, including acceptance of the feelings that may go with the hurts that drove them home. Okimoto and Stegall summarize:

> To empathize without infantilizing
> To support without controlling
> To give them what they need
> So they no longer need you.[26]

And so it may be that the welcoming home of adult children may become a very good time. Families may heal, not just the young adults. Families may carry further their unfinished business and learn how to relate lovingly to each other, adult to adult. Young adults may learn some new aspects of their parents' love for them and willingness to be there for them.

Then there will come that day for the happiness-sadness, the joyous grief of letting ago all over again.

Build a climate of mutual "friendship plus" for the rest of your lives. In my research, I came upon a term that struck me as odd. Some authorities speak of "postparental adults." In my opinion, if a person has ever been a parent, there is no such thing as being postparental! When my children had become young adults, it occurred to me that parents of young adults know something other parents do not yet know. Other parents may think that there is an end to parenting! Zenith Henkin Gross catches up this truth in the title of her study of mothers and their adult children. She titles her book *And You Thought It Was All Over!*

Her discovery is that through all the issues we have explored and beyond them, there is a long period of time with a profound relationship between parents and children. It is often sought as much on the children's initiative as on the parents'. This parenting of adult children is falsely thought by many "experts" to be virtually nonexistent. It did not exist in previous generations nearly to the extent it does today. This was due in part to the shorter life span of our parents and grandparents.

This post-launch, second-stage parenting is new to our generation and different from any of our parenting tasks before it. One mother that Gross interviewed put it this way, "At birth, they're sort of an achievement, a success. From then on until they leave home, it's responsibility—big and heavy, probably the heaviest I'll ever know. But now, it's much more carefree, much more like the pure pleasure you have with friends for whose lives you are not so responsible."[27]

I asked a number of parents of young adult children how their relationship with these offspring had changed. These are some of their answers: "We are more sensitive to each other. . . . We relate as affectionate adults. . . . We have grown in mutual respect. . . . My son has grown less dependent, and that feels good. . . . My children and I are more open and honest with each other. . . . We have learned to relate as adult to adult. . . . One of my children is following in my vocational footsteps, and that is exciting."

These parents speak of a reality that Gross and her subjects tried to define. Some called it friendship. Others said that it was simply what family was meant to be. Others called it friendship plus. It is friendship with extra bonds and extra commitments, but also extra barriers.

Gross notes at least three barriers to being friends with one's children: (1) there are not many examples of this from previous generations; (2) friendship between the generations is problematical for many reasons, primarily because age difference feeds the dependence/independence conflict; (3) the relationship has a history of one person being strong and authoritative and the other being small and responsible to the other.[28]

In the light of these barriers, these friendships are all the more surprising. Parents and children move on to a new stage of relationship with each other. (According to a character in an Ashleigh Brilliant cartoon, "I don't care what the world knows, so long as my mother doesn't find out!") In this second-stage parenting, parents and children share much more of themselves and their struggles—if not all of it. They also allow the other the right and responsibility to solve their everyday issues.

Many parents and children want a frequency of contact that may surprise some. Gross discovered that the average frequency of contact between mothers she interviewed and their adult children was once a week. (Many of the contacts were by phone, but others were made in writing or by personal visit.)

The friendship-plus stage marks the growth from dependence, to independence, to rich interdependence. It also includes the commitment of being there for each other in crisis or tragedy, to a degree that few others will share. One parent speaks of a "gut bond" that holds you together in times of tragedy. Consider the example of Barbara Timm, midlife mother of a twenty-year-old American hostage imprisoned in Iran some years ago. She traveled to Teheran against her government's orders. After a tearful confrontation with the Iranian militants guarding the United States embassy, they allowed Mrs. Timm an hour's reunion with her son.[29] Others may not have crises quite as dramatic to test parental commitment, but will respond with equally lavish concern.

Not every parent-child bond will be as close or ideal as we have described. Some may have a good bit more to overcome. And some may have much to forgive.

Still, every parent of young adults knows that a possibility exists. The possibility is of a mutual bond of friendship plus. This is something that can enrich folks who have a long history, as they share mutual growth and discovery over many years.

For Personal or Group Reflection and Discussion

1. If you have children, what was your age when they were born? What were the advantages and disadvantages of parenting at those ages?

2. What are they ages of your children now? How would you describe each of their central issues or concerns? In which of these issues is your aid as a parent welcome? In which does the child want to work it out for himself or herself?

3. Have you experienced your children's reaching out for autonomy? What forms does it take with your children? What are your wisest strategies for responding? What do you wish you had handled differently?

4. Which of the tasks of moving from childhood to adulthood were most easily accomplished by your children? Which were the most difficult?

5. Evaluate the suggestions given for responding to the range of requests, from asking for money to requests for staying home or returning home.

6. What do you celebrate in your relationship with your children? What, if you could, would you like to improve in your relationship with your children?

Resources

Coburn, Karen Levin, and Madge Lawrence Treeger. *Letting Go: A Parents' Guide to Today's College Experience.* Bethesda, Md.: Adler and Adler, 1988.

Gross, Zenith Henkin. *And You Thought It Was All Over!* New York: St. Martin's/Marek, 1985.

Levinson, Daniel, Charlotte N. Darrow, Edward B. Klein, Maria H. Levinson, and Braxton McKee. *The Seasons of a Man's Life.* New York: Alfred A. Knopf, 1978.

Newman, Barbara M., and Philip R. Newman. *Development through Life: A Psychosocial Approach.* Homewood, Ill.: The Dorsey Press, 1979.

Okimoto, Jean Davies, and Phyllis Jackson Stegall. *Boomerang Kids: How to Live with Adult Children Who Return Home.* Boston: Little, Brown, 1987.

Olson, Richard P., and Helen E. Froyd. *Discoveries: Expanding Your Child's Vocational Horizon.* Cleveland: United Church Press, 1995.

Otto, Luther B. *How to Help Your Child Choose a Career.* New York: M. Evans and Company, 1984.

Schenk, Quentin F., and Emmy Lou Schenk. *Pulling Up Roots.* Englewood Cliffs, N.J.: Prentice-Hall, 1978.

Yarrow, Andrew L. *Latecomers: Children of Parents Over 35.* New York: Free Press, 1991.

7

Caring for
Our Parents

A s we noted, the middle years often bring change to two important sets of relationships. In this chapter, we will look at the second of those—our relationship with our parents as they live with the issues of aging.

Many adults experience good health, vigor, and mobility well into old age. My mother was one of those. Into her seventies and eighties, she enjoyed life greatly. When I'd call to check about a time to come for a few days' visit, I'd often discover she wouldn't be at home because she had travel plans herself! When I did succeed in finding a time to come visit, she always had fresh-baked cinnamon rolls and chocolate chip cookies (two of her "trademarks") ready for me. I'd offer to take her out to dinner, but she'd invariably insist she'd rather cook for me. Sometimes I'd feel guilty that I didn't do more or make more regular contact, but she seemed to feel that our style of being in touch was just fine.

Near the end of her eighty-seventh year, she wrote what a wonderful year it had been. She had had a good long visit with my sister and brother-in-law in Maine, with a chance to see my sister's children and grandchildren. She had traveled to California for a celebration with foster children. Also she had been in my home in Kansas for my ordination anniversary, an event that had included my children and grandchildren. Mom commented on what a privilege it was to be able to travel and to spend time with all the persons most important to her. I lived into my fifty-fifth year without undue concern for her.

All that changed in her eighty-eighth year with a fall and a broken hip. For the rest of her life—nearly two years—her needs became massive. I will tell you a bit about that in the next chapter, and I will reflect on insights from the experience later in this one.

It will be that way with many older people. While most people would prefer to live a vigorous life until the day they die, it is not often so. Gradually or suddenly, an older person will come to need more from others.

These increased needs can occur over a range of time. And so, concerns about aging parents may come to us at any point in our middle third of life—or before it, or after it. There are a few people who discover that caring for an aging parent is one of their retirement tasks. When I surveyed numbers of people in their fifties I asked a question about their parents. I discovered that roughly one-third had already lost their parents to death; one-third were not experiencing major needs or difficulties; and one-third had elderly parents who needed much attention and care.

In this chapter we will attempt two tasks. First, we will take note of possible needs of our aging parents. Second, we will seek shared wisdom about midlife children's involvement in their parents' lives.

Needs of Our Aging Parents

Aging brings with it a variety of hazards and challenges. Older persons and their caregivers are wise to recognize these challenges and to spend time deciding how to address them. Health, mobility, memory, and safety all become key concerns, and these lead to still others.

HEALTH

A primary issue is that one's resistance to health hazards decreases and, therefore, one's susceptibility to a number of illnesses and conditions increases. A person who has lived life with a minimum of medical care may need a large amount of attention. Dr. Richard Besdine, a geriatric physician, has noted, "People . . . can fall through the cracks. . . . The problem is that many elderly do not report their illnesses. They feel that if they are old, then being sick is normal. . . . The later the intervention with the elderly, the more difficult the recuperation."[1]

Helen MacLean has listed some of the common health problems of the aging. One of these is *arteriosclerosis*, the hardening and narrowing of the arteries of the leg, resulting in circulatory impairment. There is also *atherosclerosis*, a narrowing, or clogging of coronary arteries, increasing risk of heart disease.

A frequent complaint is *arthritis*, resulting in aching joints. This cannot be cured, but can be treated so that pain is at least reduced. Closely related is *osteoarthritis*, which is joint inflammation. Prescribed exercises, pain relief, and sometimes, joint replacement are possible responses.

Emphysema, lung disease due to the destruction of tiny air sacs in the lungs, is more frequently found among persons who have been long-term heavy smokers, but is by no means confined to them.

Hearing loss may occur because of conduction deafness, which is caused by damage to some part of the middle ear, or because of nerve deafness, which comes from damage to the inner ear or the auditory nerve.

Heart failure is more accurately described as reduced heart efficiency. The heart cannot maintain normal circulation throughout the body. Medication and diet can be used to treat this condition. For some, pacemakers or bypass surgery may offered the possibility of increased vigor and added years of life.

High blood pressure (hypertension) is an indication of too much pressure against the walls of the arteries. Blood pressure includes two numbers: one records systolic pressure, which represents the pressure when the heart is contracting; the other records diastolic pressure, which represents the pressure when the heart is relaxing between beats. High blood pressure, which is without symptoms of its own, places additional strain on the aging heart, arteries, and kidneys. Proper monitoring is essential.

Malnutrition may mean not eating enough of the right foods. It may also mean eating too much of the wrong ones. For a number of reasons, older people may develop poor eating habits, which can exacerbate a variety of other health problems.

Osteoporosis is a condition in which the bones become increasingly porous, brittle, and weak. While there appears to be no single cause for this loss of bone compactness and strength, risk factors include heredity, heavy smoking, excessive use of alcohol, a low calcium-high protein diet, and lack of exercise. This condition may be one of the reasons why older people have more broken bones.

Parkinson's disease is a degenerative brain disease that affects movement, and in advanced stages, memory. There is increasing muscular rigidity, and a tremor develops, perhaps of the hands, sometimes of the head. There is no cure, but there are medications that may alleviate symptoms and minimize the progressive effects of the disease.

Vision impairment may have varied causes. Much impairment can be satisfactorily resolved by prescription eyeglasses. However some may be due to glaucoma, a fluid pressure within the eye, which must be detected early and treated regularly with eye drops to avoid permanent eye damage. Or it may be due to cataracts, in which the crystalline lens of the eye becomes cloudy. Quite frequently, these can be treated by a surgery that is quite safe.

In addition to these major diseases, there are many conditions that can make daily life uncomfortable. Some of these problems can be resolved with understanding of the cause and possibly with change in habits. Some of these "nuisance complaints" are the following: chilblains (sensitivity to cold, especially in the extremities); constipation; dental problems; dry eyes; dry mouth; fatigue; insomnia; and ringing in the ears.[2]

MacLean notes yet one other health problem that may come with aging—alcohol abuse. Persons who were never problem drinkers before may gradually use more alcohol when they have to cope with the stresses of aging. A means of coping with a problem can, in the end, become a problem itself.[3]

Increased and careful medical attention for a wide variety of possible needs is essential in older years. This needs to be done by health care professionals with sensitivity to the issues of older persons.

MEMORY AND MIND

Older people may develop serious memory lapses, physical disorientation, and/or inability to express themselves in a coherent manner. If so, they may be suffering from one of the diseases causing dementia. Though persons often use the term "Alzheimer's disease" for these problems, that may not be an accurate diagnosis.

There are many causes for failure of memory and mental functioning. Some of these causes may be reversible. Among these are the following: toxic reactions to use of barbiturates, alcohol, or multiple drug use; metabolic disorders; nutritional disorders; infection; systemic illness or disorders; and structural causes (cerebral tumors, etc.). Nonreversible dementias can be due to: Alzheimer's disease; multiple infarcts; Parkinson's disease; progressive supranuclear palsy; Huntington's disease; multiple sclerosis; AIDS; infectious diseases such as syphilis; Down's syndrome, and quite possibly others.[4] Authorities warn that misdiagnosis is all too likely. Careful evaluation is necessary to determine whether the problem is treatable and reversible, or not.

The symptoms of dementia include memory impairment; language impairment; inability to perform purposeful movement (and therefore to care for oneself); perceptual impairment; loss of ability to learn (due to the impairment of short-term memory); disorientation as to place, time, and significant persons; personality changes, most typically outbreaks of anger or rage; wandering; suspicion, delusions, and paranoia; and possible hallucinations and misinterpretations.[5]

The frequency of this family of diseases has been variously estimated. Probably somewhere between 2.5 to 6 million Americans are affected by them. Though these are by no means solely illnesses of the elderly, they do increase with age. It is estimated that dementia diseases touch one in twenty people over age sixty-five and one in five over age eighty.

One cannot overstate the tragedy of a dementia illness, both for the person who has it and for that person's family and caregivers. It is a disease that has many victims. There is an ongoing process of loss and separation for all concerned. Those caring for the person lose the person while she or he is still physically present. While it is a grieving process, the grieving is experienced again and again.

Dr. Judah Ronch tells of working with a Mrs. Molly Gruber, a former storekeeper whose functioning had become so impaired that she had been placed in a skilled nursing care facility. In that facility, she was constantly searching through others' belongings, and this was making other residents and staff quite angry. Ronch discovered Molly once spoke three languages. Though she had lost use of English, she could still speak in one of the other languages. And so he conversed with her in that language. The following is part of their interview:

> Counselor: Molly, I understand that you walk around this place all day, and go into other people's rooms. The nurses say that you look through other people's closets and drawers. Can you tell me why you do this?
>
> Mrs. Gruber: I look for Molly and I can't find her. I used to be able to read and enjoy myself, and I'd discuss what I had read with other people. But now I read and don't remember. That's not me, not the real Molly. So I walk around looking for Molly, but she's nowhere to be found.[6]

Ronch feels this expresses the heart of many person's concerns as they sense this disease coming upon them. Loss of control may be the dominating feeling. For family and friends, loss of the afflicted person may be the matching feeling.

The course of the illness varies from person to person. Some may experience it quite gradually, over a period of thirty years or more. Others may progressively experience the symptoms in just a few years. Some persons may retain characteristics, gifts, skills of an earlier time—such as Molly's language of childhood, a musical skill, etc. Others will not. Some caregivers have experienced an occasional "breakthrough" of brief but significant communication, and others have not. Each person's experience and each family's corresponding grief will be a unique story. Marion Roach, daughter of an Alzheimer's patient, has written:

> It goes on and on, and just when we can't stand one phase, we don't have to, because it's succeeded by another one—a worse phase, a more outrageous phase, a quieter phase, a sloppier phase, a more confused phase, a phase of hushed panic—seen in the eyes of the victim, seen by us.[7]

Those who care for persons with dementia disease are in extremely high stress situations. They need much rest, respite, and support.

Many persons have a much smaller degree of memory loss. Short-term memory loss may mean that one may forget to turn off the stove or iron. At this stage, it is difficult to know whether one can safely live independently and alone—the way of life many older adults prefer.

LIFE TASKS

The issues we have spoken of lead to others. With increased health problems and medical needs, and with decreased mobility and strength, everyday life tasks become more demanding.

The obtaining and preparing of food takes a larger proportion of energy. Making and keeping medical appointments may be difficult. Remembering to take an increasingly complicated set of medications may be overwhelming.

Persons who once took great pride in the care of their home and yard may not have energy left over to do it. One of my midlife friends visited her parents during a Christmas vacation. These were people who used to decorate their home beautifully; that year, they had managed to drag out their artificial tree and hang one string of forlorn lights on it. Such was the energy they had for a task that once was easy and a joy.

Self-care may also be neglected. Personal hygiene, laundering and ironing of clothes, attention to appearance may demand too much of one.

In many communities, there are services that will help older people with these issues. Many resist, either because they don't want strangers in their home or because of cost. Still, they may need to be vigorously encouraged to use such services to maintain a quality of life. They may need to be encouraged to name what services will contribute to their enjoyment of life. I remember how much my mother delighted in the hair wash and curling that a volunteer did for her weekly in the hospital.

MOBILITY

In our society especially, many enjoy the freedom that comes with owning and driving a car. It allows a spontaneity about decisions of where to go and when.

Still, the time may come when older persons need to give up this privilege and responsibility. The most frequent reason is a loss of vision. Slower reaction times are another problem. This creates a hazard both for the driver and for others. It is a sad and somber day when one fails the vision part of a relicensing test. For some this event has sapped the enthusiasm for living.

One midlife person saw another reason why her parent should discontinue driving. Her father, who was in the mid-stages of Parkinson's disease, would go out driving. Occasionally he would forget where he parked the car!

Adult children of older persons may need to face this issue with parents and to devise other ways of assuring their parents' mobility. One person discovered that it was possible to make an agreement with a taxi company, which included making a deposit of money. It proved to provide great freedom of safe, worry-free movement and was less costly than the maintenance and insurance on a car.

SAFETY

The same environment in which one flourished at an early age may become unsafe in one's older years.

Dark passages; steep steps; stairs and bathrooms without handrails; throw rugs, stools, or low tables over which one may trip—all of these and more may be dangerous for an older person. They may need safety measures taken in existing housing, or they may need to move to smaller, one-level housing facilities that offer a greater chance of safety from accidents. Bright lights may need to be added.

Weather may bring safety hazards as well. Ice, snow, sleet, rain can make surfaces slippery and dangerous. Older people may need to hire someone to clear sidewalks and may also need to lay in extra supplies against inclement weather.

Older people may live in neighborhoods that have become physically hazardous. One elderly couple liked their home, neighborhood, and community church. They hated to think of leaving. However, the increase of violent crime in that area held them in constant dread and fear. A midlife daughter persuaded them to move out of the neighborhood—indeed, to move several hundred miles and find housing close to her. "They were so relieved," she recalls, "I saw them shed ten years of age in just a few months."

FREEDOM FROM HARASSMENT

Regrettably, unscrupulous persons sometimes take advantage of older people.

One midlife woman, in going over her grandmother's checkbook, discovered that she had been making regular payments on an insurance policy. Looking at the policy, the woman discovered it had no relevance to her grandmother's needs. The grandmother confessed she really didn't want it, but found herself unable to say no to a persistent, argumentative salesman.

In my interviews, I learned of an even more tragic situation. A midlife person went to see her mother, a woman who had been quite independent and had managed her finances quite well. The daughter discovered that her mother was destitute. She had sent some money to a religious broadcaster, whose representatives had called again and again, insisting on more gifts, until she had given everything she had away. She was unable to provide even for her own needs as she had always intended.

It is difficult to be aware of every person who might harass older folks for financial gain. However, it is important to be aware that it happens and be sensitive to any signs of its occurring.

HUMAN DIGNITY, SELF-DETERMINATION, AND COMMUNITY

There is another family of needs, perhaps even more important but not as easily catalogued and described as those above. I refer to the need for human dignity in the face of the indignities of aging, and the need for those things that make life worth living.

Perhaps at the top of the list of these is the need for self-determination. At very least, one wants to be involved in the decisions about one's future. These decisions may be complex and confusing. They may be hedged by practical concerns such as limited finances. Yet, the older person needs to express what he or she wants and have it honored as much as possible.

In such conversations, I have seen some midlife persons and their parents come to the conclusion that the parents will move near to their children. That way, the children can give more constant watchful care and attention. Other midlife children and their parents have decided that the parents should stay in their community, even though it means the children can provide less direct care.

These decisions will be based on what the parents hold most dear in living. What will they give up most reluctantly? These persons may want to live out their days among their lifelong friends. Their Sunday school class or other groups at church may provide a vital fellowship. They may feel comfortable with merchants, health care providers, eating places, and other things that make their present community their desired one.

Another area of needed sensitivity is that older persons may move, talk, think, and decide more slowly. Persons working with them should take time to come to conclusions with which the older persons can live. When I lived at a distance from my mother and could come only occasionally for a brief visit, this was hard for me to remember. I wanted to be helpful and assist her in making decisions about needed care. At times my time pressures made me less sensitive to my mother's need for time to ponder these decisions.

Lest we fall into the trap of thinking of older parents only as a burden, another perspective needs to be added. Many cultures revere older people. They seek the advice and wisdom of the elderly and hold it in extremely high regard. We will do well to approach these tasks and decisions anticipating our parents' wisdom, not only about what is best for them but about many other matters as well.

Our Responses as Midlife Children

We have outlined some of the needs of aging parents. Now, what fitting response should we midlife children make? These are the people who gave us birth, raised us, and lent interest and support to this day. What response shall we make as age and frailty increase?

DO NOT BUY INTO A HARMFUL MYTH

If a parent becomes frail and needy, the midlife person needs a clear awareness of the new situation and new roles in which parent and child find themselves. In this connection, Mark Edinberg points out that there is a rather harmful myth in the making. That is the myth of "parenting the parent" or "role reversal." He points out that even though adult children of the elderly may become advisers, care providers, and sources of emotional and financial support to their parents, they are not their parents' parents. This is a misleading and problematical way to describe the situation.

The parent is not a child, even if there are childlike needs or behaviors to consider. Further, the caregiver's task is not to "raise" one's parents, but rather to help them cope and adapt to the losses that life is bringing them.

Edinberg tells of working with Rosa, a sixty-eight-year-old woman dying of cancer, and her daughter Kay. Rosa needed help walking and was also incontinent, wearing adult diapers.

Kay began to talk about how their situation had "reversed," how now she was the "parent" and her mother was the "child." I watched Kay's discomfort play itself out on her face and body, and was also aware that Rosa was crying silently. . . . I said the following: "Kay, you are not her mother; she is not your child. Even if you are changing Rosa's diapers because she is incontinent, even if you are helping her walk, you are both adults. You can do all of these things and still be Rosa's adult daughter." I watched both of them relax as I spoke. Each, it appeared, was glad to be freed from the bind of having the daughter "parent the parent."[8]

FACE AND WORK OUT YOUR RESISTANCES

Consider the following story. Long ago, a farmer knew that his father, who had reached the then ripe old age of seventy, was no longer productive. And so he sent him out to the barn to live—a condition where the old man would quite likely die soon from lack of food and from exposure. In one act of compassion, the farmer told his son to bring the old man a meager blanket to cover him. Shortly the son returned, carrying half of the blanket. The farmer was upset at this and asked, "Why did you leave that old man with just half a blanket to cover him?" The son replied, "Father, I saved some of the blanket for you."[9]

The story reminds us that we have a self-interest in seeing to it that the elderly are well treated. It also points to the complicated dynamics that make it difficult for us to think straight and act responsibly with our parents. We may resist because we find it hard to think about our own aging, much less that of our parents. Their frailty is an all too potent reminder that ours is coming. Or we may find it hard to think of not having them as a firm foundation and source of family strength.

We may resist because we find the responsibility overwhelming. It may appear simply endless, and we don't know how to be involved without being overwhelmed.

Some of us may resist because of unresolved pain with our parents. There may be ongoing personality conflicts or memories of painful encounters. For some there may be even memories of physical, emotional, or sexual abuse.

Whatever the sources of our resistance, they need to be faced and worked on. Possibly other family members or good friends can hear out one's agony. A therapist's help may be needed.

It will be helpful to all if we are clear in our minds about these resistances. Each person may need to decide what he or she is willing and able to do with/for his or her parents in the light of such feelings. Unexamined, resisting, resentful half responses or nonresponses are not good for anyone.

AS MUCH AS YOU CAN, PLAN RATHER THAN REACT

Tom Koch was a midlife person who returned home and cared for his father, Norman, through the last several months of his life as he suffered through a protracted geriatric illness. Koch wrote the story of that care and what his family learned from it in the book *Mirrored Lives: Aging Children and Elderly Parents.* He recalls how fulfilling it was to give this care to his father in the early stages:

> Tiring though it was for me, I enjoyed those early weeks. The loyalty and love I felt for Father, emotions that had never been expressed before, now had a focus and outlet. He had always insisted on being in charge, the one who offered aid but would accept nothing in return. This was my chance to repay that debt by bringing him back to a strength and purpose he had once given me.[10]

However, as the months wore on, there was increasing tension. He could have borne the exertion of this task (with occasional time away). What he found troubling was the developing tensions and disagreements between father and children, and among the children themselves. This was occurring in a family that loved each other, had a rich family history, and ordinarily dealt with each other rather well.

Koch identified four areas of serious disagreement between his father and him (along with his brothers). These were home care, financial planning, legal arrangements, and liaison with medical practitioners. In each of these areas his father increasingly felt diminished, enfeebled, and losing control.

While some of this tension was probably an inevitable part of a protracted illness, in retrospect Koch felt they could have reduced the problems considerably. However, they would have had to do one important but difficult task: They would have had to anticipate and plan, rather than react. He feels they did not prepare because they refused to accept the possibility of a protracted geriatric illness.

If they faced that possibility, together they could have done some planning, though it would be impossible to anticipate every contingency. But they could have been more attuned to each other's concerns and questions, and to their father's preferences for home care, medical treatment, extraordinary measures, and more.

Koch tells of a friend who learned from his experience. This friend, Paul C., was worried about the declining health of his parents. Paul lived close to his parents, and his only brother lived at some distance. When his brother was visiting, Paul decided to introduce these topics. He recalls,

> I was kind of nervous at first, but my father said he and mother had thought about these issues a lot and knew what they wanted. My brother said how he felt and what he'd do, and I said what if one parent gets sick and the other can't take care? We talked for hours, and at the end I knew I wasn't alone [in my fears] and wouldn't be alone if something happened.[11]

Clearly, neither of these families could plan everything about the parents' geriatric needs. They could open the topic and begin to lay the foundation for future mutual discussion.

There is yet another area that needs family discussion and pre-planning. This has to do with "extraordinary" measures in health care. Which treatments are wanted and which are not desired when a person's health has become very frail and quality of life is not what it used to be? There are at least two points of decision. In the event of cardiac failure, does one want to be resuscitated, and, possibly, put on a ventilator to aid breathing? If not, one can ask one's physician to put a DNR—Do not resuscitate—order on one's medical records. The other is, does one want to be fed by a feeding tube if one is unable to take nourishment by mouth? If so, does one want the right to determine when to stop this procedure? These matters should also be discussed with one's physician. Quite probably, they should also be registered both through a Living Will and a Durable Power of Attorney for Health Care. Copies of these documents should be placed with one's physician, attorney, family caregiver, possibly with one's minister, and any other significant caregivers. We will discuss these documents in more detail in the next chapter.

These decisions about health care—DNR, Living Will, Durable Power of Attorney for Health Care—should be registered at the hospital at every admission. It is unlikely that such information will carry over automatically from a previous admission.

SHARE DECISION MAKING—SHARE RESPONSIBILITIES

One expression of the principle stated above—that a frail parent is still an adult, not a child—will come into play in decisions about that person's place to live, care, and treatment. Slow, careful discussion, carried on in advance of emergencies, will serve well. There needs to be honesty and frankness—sometimes mid-adult children are unable to fulfill their parents' preferences. However, respect for those wishes and attempts to concur are basic. These wishes need to be known by all adult children and any others who may be involved in the care of the elderly person.

There also needs to be discussion about how responsibilities will be shared. Too often, the greatest responsibility falls on one person. Are there ways that this can be more justly shared? Tom Koch describes one division that, he feels, would have served their family well.

He suggests having a clear sense of the range of responsibilities that go with providing care and community for an elderly person. Then these responsibilities can be divided and delegated. A person may accept more than one of them—perhaps one person will need to do virtually all of them. Still, clarity about the range of needs and of conscious efforts to respond will be helpful.

Out of his experience and conversations with others, he identifies at least six roles that are areas of concern:

1. *Primary Caregiver.* This is the individual whose task is the daily medical and home maintenance of the older person. Someone needs to be in touch and concerned about these matters, whether the older person is at home or in a nursing home. This person will need relief from time to time, but others should defer to this person's decisions and judgments about care.

2. *Financial Surrogate.* The financial caretaker should discuss with the older person the broad outline of that person's financial picture before illness strikes. This person can be aware of the range of resources and how the older person wants them used, should the need arise.

3. *Legal Surrogate.* This person would learn from the older person about his or her legal affairs—Who is the attorney? Where are legal documents stored? What financial institutions are used? Is there a will and, if so, who has a copy? What medical insurance does the person hold? A person who has been made knowledgeable about these matters and is authorized to act when needed will be most helpful.

4. *Medical Surrogate.* Koch, in looking back, wished deeply that he had accompanied his father on at least one visit to his father's physician before his father became so ill. At that time, his father could have told the physician that in the event of severe illness, this son would be vitally involved, would participate in decisions, was entitled to any medical information the family needed. Even without that prior arrangement, it is wise to have one designated person—who has the family's confidence—to converse and negotiate with health care providers.

5. *Community Surrogate.* Tom Koch, on reflection, realized his family had failed to utilize an important resource, his father's peers and other community persons. And so he suggests a community surrogate. Some of this close circle of associates saw the health problems coming before the family did. These persons also made convalescence easier. Yet it was not clear how family caregivers and community friends should collaborate for this person's welfare. A person giving attention to this could rally these community resources and let them know when, where, and how to be encouraging and helpful.

6. *Relations Surrogate.* Extended family, probably spread over many miles, is also concerned. And so Koch suggests a relations surrogate. This person can keep the relatives informed and let them know how they can lend support. This person may also need to enforce one unbending rule—no second-guessing the persons who are present, giving care, and making decisions.[12]

There may be need to be discussion of financial provision for the person who handles the primary caregiver role, and probably much more. This caregiving is a sacrifice, even if freely offered. The caregiver may need to interrupt other employment. Families need to learn to respond and support each other fittingly.

Other families may divide the care tasks differently. For example, I know of one family where the daughter who lived in the same community provided the bulk of the care needed. Other family members were sensitive to her needs for time away from this responsibility. They came in to spell her so that she could have needed weekends away, as well as vacations and holidays with her children.

Families also need to discover what services may need to be contracted with community care providers. In many areas, a wide range of services are available for families that don't have the personnel, expertise, or time to do them all. Housekeeping, meals, nursing, physical therapy, and more may be available in one's own home. Adult day care may provide a safe environment, together with stimulating activities, people contact, and a nutritious meal. Persons are brought back to their own homes for the evening and overnight.

There are residential complexes that provide a range of housing and care needs for elderly persons. Sometimes if persons are admitted to one aspect—a small apartment with a daily meal, for example—they have access to the skilled care facilities should they need them later.

Many older persons dread and resist the idea of ever entering a "nursing home." It may sound like a sentence for diminished life, joyless living, and imminent death. For some convalescent homes of the past and present, that might have been an accurate appraisal, yet much is changing in this field. And, for some, this may be a necessary decision to see that an older parent is provided the safe care and supervision needed. This hard decision will be softened if it is discussed in advance. The family may need to explore such facilities and options within them, difficult as this is. Visits to and frank discussions with friends using these facilities may help clarify the questions. Many of the good facilities have waiting lists. People may wait months or years to be admitted. Perhaps a first step can be made by putting a name on a waiting list in a nonbinding, "just in case" scenario.

APPROPRIATE YOUR FAMILY HISTORY, LEGACY, WISDOM

It's time to complete your "family business." Within one's living parents, there resides a knowledge of family history and of the human legacy of one's family. Some will have a more vivid awareness of this knowledge than others. Some treasure it, while others tend to ignore and forget it. Some speak freely of it, while others need to have this information coaxed out of them.

One knows oneself most completely if one knows one's family history and heritage. And so, quite possibly, aging parents have a valuable gift for those who will listen and accept: the gift of family memories. They may also have documents, other written information, and pictures of previous generations as well. (If so, do you know where this information is? Is it labeled so that you know what you are seeing? Is there clarity and more perspective to be gained by inviting your parents to talk about those pictures, documents, genealogies, etc.?)

I came to desire this kind of information almost too late. Then, I needed to be more skillful than I was in eliciting it from my mom. I remember a time that I failed miserably. Filled with enthusiasm for "oral history" I came in like "gang busters" on one visit, complete with tape recorder and many blank tapes. I use tape recorders almost daily and am quite comfortable with them. My mother was not. The tape recorder intimidated and frightened her. She clammed up. "I don't know what you want," she told me repeatedly. We dropped it for that trip.

A few years later, when she was confined to a hospital bed, I asked some of the same questions, much more gently, in a relaxed and quiet manner—and without the tape recorder. Somehow that stirred a willingness to reminisce that she had not often shared with me. I learned things I never knew about my maternal grandmother, about my mother and father's courtship, engagement, and marriage. We were interrupted several times by visitors, but when they left, each time she would return to those memories we had been talking about. At the end of the day, she told me how much she had enjoyed our conversations.

I was not prepared for the huge amount of memory and information my mom shared. Lacking a notebook, I jotted down things on every piece of scrap paper I could find. Shortly after I returned home, I typed out my summary of everything she told me. There were gaps in it—things I forgot to ask, names she mentioned that I couldn't remember. I sent her a copy of this, hoping it would stimulate further remembering.

On my next visit, a month or so later, I asked her if she received that information. She said yes, and then asked me where I got all that. "From you," I responded. She looked at me strangely, and showed no further inclination to discuss those things.

Other relatives did fill in some of the gaps. I am grateful for all the family heritage I gleaned before my mother's death. Yet, even now I wish I knew more. For example, Mom passed on a lovely piece of furniture—a curved-glass china cabinet—to my wife, Mary Ann. I half-know the story: it was given to Mom with the proviso that when she could no longer use it, she would give it to a minister's wife. But who gave it to her, and when, and why was that a condition? I didn't think to ask, and now I probably will never know.

Perhaps my experience will trigger an interest in you. If your parents and/or other aged relatives are living, think about it. How well do you know your family heritage? Do you know it both in the broad strokes—nationalities, names, occupations, size of families—as well as in the delicate nuances—strengths and weaknesses, ways of caring for each other, ways of doing conflict? Are there beloved family stories that you would like to get down the way they have been told? Is there information about genealogy that they may know how to access but you don't? Gaining this more complete picture and the experience of receiving it from your parents may be something you will treasure.

For some, there may also be a negative side to this. There may be "family business" that needs to be completed. I am not speaking of finances, loans, or bequests, but the business of living with each other. Some may feel let down by parents, hurt by parents, hampered by parents. Persons may be adult children of alcoholics, past or present. There may be memories with unforgiven aspects that may flow either or both ways.

In order to be more healthy, the midlife person may need to face these issues and reach some resolution. Sometimes parents can participate in these healings and reconciliations, sometimes not. At the very least, seeing one's parents in the light of *their* history and heritage may lend perspective.

Sometime in midlife years, one awakens to the fact that there is limited time to do some important things. That is, to collect and appropriate one's family history, and to complete, as much as possible, any unfinished family transactions.

RECOGNIZE THAT THE TASK IS TO CARE RATHER THAN TO CURE

Henri Nouwen has noted that when one is offering aid to the elderly, it is important to know what one is doing. There is, he suggests, a difference between the motive of *cure* and the motive of *care*.

Ours is a society with great emphasis on cure. Fix it, make it better, preferably as quickly as possible. That is wonderful—when it works. And it works, sometimes, with the injuries, surgeries, and illnesses of the elderly.

However, there will come a time in the life of each person when there will not be a cure. Tom Koch notes, "Debilitating age is a new disease and one for which we can conceive no cure, a gradual but pervasive condition that affects us all."[13] When caring for an older person who is at that stage—she or he won't get better but only worse—that is the point where the motive of *care* becomes so important. There are those whose interest declines when it becomes obvious that no cure will be forthcoming. May it not be so among family caregivers.

Caring means to making oneself available to the experience of becoming old. It means entering into that experience. It means being a caring presence, offering what is needed, whether that is talking, listening, doing, or simply being there. It is seeing to the person beyond the limitations now imposed on him or her. It is listening for and recognizing the wisdom and courage that others may not take the time to hear. It is acceptance if one must cry, complain, talk about fears and aches and pains. Though we have no cures to offer, in caring, we may both offer and receive the greatest gifts. Nouwen writes:

> The most important contribution to the elderly is to offer them a chance to bring us into creative contact with our own aging. . . . Thus we can be brought in touch with the fullness of the life experience by an inner solidarity with all human suffering and all human growth. This inner solidarity is the basis of the human community where real care and healing can take place. Therefore we entered into the darkness so that we might come to the light, and we spoke about the aging self to come to a fuller care of the aging others.
>
> Aging is one of the most essential human processes, one that can be denied only with great harm. Every man and woman who has discovered or rediscovered his or her own aging has a unique opportunity to enrich the quality of his or her own life and that of every fellow human being.[14]

RECOGNIZE YOUR LIMITS; CARE FOR YOURSELF AS WELL AS OTHERS

The midlifer who is the prime caregiver to parents has an incredibly broad task, especially if it is coupled with simultaneous needs from his or her own children. One woman cried out,

> What's happened to me? I'm like the rope in a tug of war between my parents and my children. I always seem to be needed in two

places at the same time and I'm never in the right one. . . . It's aw-
ful to feel so guilty all the time. But do you know there's something even worse? It's that little voice inside my head that's always
crying out, "What about me? When is there going to be time for
me? Doesn't anybody care?"[15]

If that cry for self care of which she speaks is not answered, she
will lose the capacity to do anything else. Or she may do it but as
an automaton, all feelings having been stamped out.

Every person in that circumstance may need to come to several
conclusions. For one, I have a sacred responsibility to my parents.
Family love and biblical command converge at this point. At the
same time, this responsibility is but one among several. I will not
overemphasize this one so much that I disrupt or destroy family,
or career, or self.

Again, I am vulnerable. I have needs and possible fatigue that
deserve attention. I need help and must learn to ask for it and accept it when the demands are too great.

Further, my needs for self care are legitimate, both in themselves and as the means by which I will be able to continue to give
care. Finally, I can take comfort in the fact that there is only one,
God, who neither slumbers nor sleeps. Having done all I can do, I
will trust my God, the God of my parents, to grant strength and
guidance for the rest.

As a midlifer, care for my parents is both a privilege and a responsibility. May it also be a growing time from which I emerge
without regret, with an increased sense of family, and with an acceptance of my own aging process.

For Personal or Group Reflection and Discussion

1. In your group it might be good to know where each is with
regard to parents. Are your parents reasonably healthy and self
sufficient; struggling with health and many needs; or deceased?

2. Do any in your group have parents coping with mild or severe memory loss? What steps are they taking to respond?

3. Are any members in the group engaging community resources or housing communities to provide for parental needs? How is this working out?

4. Is there some division of family responsibilities for the needs of your parents? If so, how was this decided? How is it working? Are there aspects of it that need to be renegotiated?

5. Do you recognize resistances in yourself that make it hard to be helpful to your parents? Do you recognize the source of these? How are you dealing with them?

6. Do you feel your family plans or reacts as to your parents' needs?

7. Do you know as much about your family heritage and history as you would like? If not, what else would you like to know? In what ways can your parents help you with that search?

8. How does faith and church undergird you in your care for your parents?

Resources

Burger, Sharon Greene, and Martha D'Erasmo. *Living in a Nursing Home*. New York: Ballantine Books, 1976.

Curtin, Sharon R. *Nobody Ever Died of Old Age*. Boston: Little, Brown, 1972.

Edinberg, Mark A. *Talking with Your Aging Parents*. Boston: Shambhala, 1987.

Koch, Tom. *Mirrored Lives: Aging Children and Elderly Parents*. New York: Praeger, 1990.

MacLean, Helene. *Caring for Your Parents*. Garden City, N.Y.: Doubleday, 1987.

Nouwen, Henri J. M., and Walter J. Gaffney. *Aging: The Fulfillment of Life*. Garden City, N.Y.: Image Books, 1976.

Ronch, Judah L. *Alzheimer's Disease: A Practical Guide for Those Who Help Others*. New York: Continuum, 1989.

Shulman, Bernard H., and Raeann Berman. *How to Survive Your Aging Parents*. Chicago: Surrey Books, 1988.

Silverstone, Barbara, and Helen Kandel Hyman. *You and Your Aging Parent*. New York: Pantheon Books, 1976.

Woller, Dwight Lee. *Forgiving Our Parents: For Adult Children from Dysfunctional Families*. Minneapolis: CompCare Publishers, 1989.

III

Inner
Journeys
in the
Middle Years

8

Facing Death in Myself and Those I Love

N ow THAT WE have explored many of midlife's outer tasks, it is time to turn to the inner journey. We will begin at a strange but necessary starting place—the subject of death. For all of us, at some time and in some manner, midlife brings a twofold encounter with death.

In the introduction I told you about one aspect of this for me— a dizzying, disorienting preoccupation with my own death. This occurred shortly after my fortieth birthday. In the midst of this anguish, I did not expect any relief, ever. Indeed, the diminishing of this heavy cloud of dread was so slow and gradual that I did not sense it was lifting. Very, very slowly, I realized that I wasn't as troubled over my eventual death. Though those thoughts sometimes return, they no longer have the sting they had during that troubling forty-first year of my life.

As I look back to that period of my life and those feelings, one thing strikes me as strange—I was entirely preoccupied with *me*. My inner personal dread was not matched by a look outward. I did not reflect on the fact that the people I hold dear are also mortal and that one of life's greatest pains is letting them go when they die. This was in spite of the fact that my dad had died when I was a child, and my wife Mary Ann's mother had died when we were in our twenties. At that period of time (my early forties), my self-pre-occupation crowded out past griefs and probable future ones.

Too soon my focus had to change. Though I did not die in my forties or fifties, a number of persons important to me did. We lost Mary Ann's dad and her grandmother, who had been such a loving presence in our home from time to time. As I also mentioned in the introduction, we lost our good friends Dave and Mary.

Each of these losses brought its own unique pain. In retro-spect, each also prepared me for this last year when death has taken two persons from my inner circle of greatest support. I need to tell you a little about each and about their deaths.

One of the persons I lost to death was my mother. Mom was a plucky woman. Though she had been totally unprepared to be a widow in her early forties, with two grade-school children, she had pulled herself together. She fought off the poverty, sacrificed, and encouraged our dreams. As a result of her encouragement, modeling, and giving, both my sister Ruth and I achieved the col-lege education and professional training to which we aspired. More than anyone else in all the earth, she believed in my sister and me. She was so proud of us—and our families, children, and grandchildren.

The other person was one of my two closest pals, Lee Regier. Lee and I were good friends from high-school days. We had been classmates and daily companions through college years. After we completed our graduate education, we stayed in touch in every possible way—spending time together in each other's churches and homes and at conventions. Mostly the phone was our link. We shared absolutely everything with each other. We told our secrets and did not hide our feelings. If either of us was sad, mad, or glad, we'd pick up the phone and talk it over with the other. Of all the things I treasured in Lee, most of all I loved his humor and laugh-ter. He stirred the playful child in me as no one else ever has.

Mom had enjoyed reasonably good health through her eighty-seventh year. However, in her eighty-eighth, she underwent two major surgeries, first a broken hip, and then removal of a large por-tion of her stomach. She tried valiantly to learn to walk again, and did succeed enough to be able to be in her own home—with round-the-clock care—for a brief time. However, her health problems compounded. In the winter of her eighty-ninth year, she needed more care than could be given in a private home. She was taken back to the hospital, awaiting placement in a convalescent home.

I live 430 miles from where my mom lived. As she was experiencing all of this, I would attempt to go spend a few days with her every two to three months. Though I felt bad at what she was going through, for the most part those were good visits. These times together always ended the same way—the day I left I would come in and see her first thing in the morning. Aware that if I left promptly I could be home for supper, she would thank me for coming, kiss me, and urge me out the door.

On a visit in March, it was different. That morning, she ignored the fact I needed to leave shortly. After staying as long as I felt I could, I reluctantly told her I had to go. I promised that I would return as soon as I could. She cried and hugged me closely. She clung to me and did not want to let me go. As I look back, I realize that she knew more than I and was telling me goodbye. She died two weeks later.

I felt that my grief wounds for Mom were deep but clean. Though I had lived a fair distance from her since youth, we had expressed our love for each other, and said most of the things we needed to each other. We had been there for each other. However, even if the wounds are clean, there is grief! This grief expressed itself in a number of ways. Part of it was denial. When, a few months later, I made a trip back to her community to see the people who cared for her, see her grave stone, and transact some business, I still half expected her to be there greeting me. Another aspect was anger. At times I would find myself impatient at work, or unexpectedly angry at some pettiness. Then I would realize it was my grief showing up in an unexpected place. There was and will be more expressions—unexpected or expected. I cannot (and I do not want to), lose the impact of her life and death upon me.

There were two intentional actions I undertook as part of my grief work. One was to memorialize Mom and Dad. For me, this took the form of writing. Once this need occurred to me, I called my sister Ruth, who felt the same way and entered into this project with me. (This took some doing—she lives in Maine and I live in Kansas.) Throughout summer and fall, we collected memorabilia and documents; wrote up genealogical material; put our personal memories of Mom and Dad on paper; brought to light discoveries about the healthful and unhealthful ways our family operated; and prepared charts of the marriages and children of each of our children. We added photographs, birth and marriage certificates, and other mementos. This was a healing exercise both for Ruth and for me. As her counselor said when she described the project, "It sounds like a love letter to your mom." Somehow, it felt compelling, not only to do this project but to do it at the time we did. I wanted for us to compile this in the first year after Mom died and to be able to give it as Christmas gifts to our children.

The other intentional grief response was to "do it now." I came to feel even more strongly that whatever expressions of love and support we want to express to important persons in our lives should not be delayed; they should to be expressed while they are living. One form this took was that my sister and I invited our children, children-in-law, and grandchildren to a family reunion in the lovely seaside resort community where my sister lives. Mom would have loved that event.

Another expression of this "do it now" attitude was a reunion with Lee in September. When I heard that his contributions were to be recognized with an honorary degree, I determined—along with other close friends, Ron and Marjorie Erickson—to go to California to celebrate with him. (All our lives, Lee and I had poked fun at honorary degrees. I wanted him to know that his was deserved, backed by the love and respect of many friends.) We had a wonderful time together with private parties and public celebrations—and laughter far into the night. True, even though I knew he had been having health problems, I was shocked at his ashen appearance. Unbidden, the thought had flitted across my mind that this might be our last time together. I pushed that aside and enjoyed my friends. Out of that rich time, Lee and I agreed that we needed to have closer touch and would phone each other weekly. We succeeded in doing so, most weeks.

In December, aided by computer disk and telephone, Ruth and I finished our memories-through-writing project. We called it "Roots and Wings—One Family's Story." I polished a few more pages, collected all the material together, and took it to the printer to have a dozen copies reproduced.

When I returned to my office, there was a long-distance call awaiting me. Barbara, Lee's wife, was calling to tell me that Lee had died in his sleep that morning. Scarcely had one grief wound begun to heal than another opened!

I decided that I would not travel to Lee's memorial service, but would visit Barb, his wife, and Deborah, his daughter, later. The Sunday on which his service took place was Christmas Sunday, and I had heavy commitments on that Sunday, including something Lee had taught me. Each year during Advent, Lee had planned and led a "Christmas service for the grieving." This was designed to acknowledge and lend support to those who found Christmas a difficult time because of grief pangs. I had planned such a service and was conducting it in Kansas at the very moment that Lee's memorial service was being held in California. At the end of that service, I lit a candle for Lee.

I am recalling and writing about these events some months after they occurred. While other reflections and discoveries will be shared later in this chapter, one is clear at this moment. This midlife task is twofold: facing and dealing with one's own finitude and death; facing and dealing with the loss of those one loves—either in anticipation or response. Neither issue by itself is complete. Failure to deal with one aspect inhibits one's ability to deal with the other. Conversely, finding strength to deal with one aspect may well lend strength to deal with the other. In this chapter I will share resources that will lend aid in dealing with either or both aspects of this basic task in the inner midlife pilgrimage.

What resources are available to help us face our finitude?

At this point we can benefit from the counsel of Elizabeth Kubler-Ross, the pioneer who helped us discover what the dying have to teach us. Dr. Kubler-Ross has suggested how helpful it would be if more of us would talk about death and dying as an intrinsic part of life, just as we freely discuss birth. If we did this, it would be a much more simple task to help a patient deal with a terminal illness, she says.[1] She prefers discussing death and dying with patients long before it actually happens, if the patient indicates a readiness for that. In her opinion, "a healthier, stronger individual can deal with it better and be less frightened by oncoming death when it is still 'miles away' than when it is 'right in front of the door.'"[2]

Well, we are presumably "miles away" from our own and other persons' deaths, but they are coming. Living is a terminal situation. Quite possibly, during teenage and early adult years, the major developmental tasks (identity, intimacy, etc.) are so heavy that persons *have* to repress the dilemma of death in order to get the other tasks worked out. But now in the middle years the time in life has come really to "look" at death, to "unrepress" that dreaded but important subject.

But how does one do that? When one speaks of death, one describes (in theologian Paul Tillich's terms) an "existential anxiety," not a "neurotic anxiety." This death anxiety cannot be removed by pills or positive thinking or psychoanalysis.

Still, there are steps that can be taken to deal with death anxiety. Consider the terms "unrepress," "deal with," "work out"—a term that brings to mind the Bible verses, "[W]ork out your own salvation with fear and trembling; for it is God who is at work in you . . ." (Phil. 2:12–13)—or "grief work." These terms imply that one need not remain immobilized by panic. A person can face this issue. One can absorb its truth down into the depth of one's being. Then one can also sense community with other persons and their support in this dilemma. These are ultimately steps of faith in our Source.

I want to assist in this process of raising consciousness, stimulating discussion, and helping each person examine attitudes. Let's explore six aspects of this topic: (1) the nature and experience of loss; (2) the stages of dying and lessons from this for midlife persons; (3) the range of choices one has regarding one's dying; (4) the ways we seek and claim immortality; (5) what the dying and those who have been near death have to teach us; (6) a Christian perspective on these matters.

The Nature and Experience of Loss

Kenneth R. Mitchell and Herbert Anderson developed some important insights on loss in their book, *All Our Losses, All Our Griefs*. They point out that while loss due to the death of a loved person is relatively rare, loss is constant throughout life. In some ways these losses are "little deaths," anticipatory deaths. The experience of loss and the methods we develop for coping with loss will influence us in many ways. They will impact how we respond to the deaths of others and how we react to the foreknowledge of our own death.

Mitchell and Anderson discovered that there are at least six major types of loss.

1. *Material Loss.* "Material loss is the loss of a physical object or of familiar surroundings to which one has an important attachment."[3] An object may be valued because of its origin—for example, it may have been a gift from a beloved person. Or it may be valued because of some quality of its own. Loss of a prized object, the necessity of moving from a familiar and loved place, and (perhaps) the death of a pet, are some examples of material loss. Many persons are introduced to grief through the death of a pet. Outsiders may not realize how deep the pain of that grief is!

2. *Relationship Loss.* "Relationship loss is the ending of opportunities to relate oneself to, talk with, share experiences with, make love to, touch, settle issues with, fight with, and otherwise be in the emotional and/or physical presence of a particular other human being."[4] Moving away (or a friend's moving), a summer vacation, divorce, widowhood are all examples. Relationship loss may be mild or severe, temporary or permanent, but it comes to every person.

3. *Intrapsychic Loss.* "Intrapsychic loss is the experience of losing an emotionally important image of oneself, losing the possibilities of 'what might have been,' abandonment of plans for a particular future, the dying of a dream. Although often related to external experiences, it is

itself an entirely inward experience."[5] A person may recognize that one does not have the talent or will not have the opportunity to pursue a dream. One might complete a task and need to move on. A person may be promoted and removed from treasured tasks and colleagues. All of these might be intrapsychic losses.

4. *Functional Loss.* "Powerful grief can be evoked when we lose some of the muscular or neurological functions of the body."[6] One may lose sight, or hearing, or coordination. Along with this, one may lose mobility and autonomy. A person may lose long-term or short-term memory. Anger or touchiness when such change of function is brought up may well be a normal grief reaction to such loss.

5. *Role Loss.* "The loss of a specific social role or of one's accustomed place in a social network is experienced as role loss."[7] Retirement, being promoted, going back to school, entering a hospital as patient are all examples of role loss and role change. In each, there may be a grief process that is marked, at least in part, by disorientation.

6. *Systemic Loss.* People live in "interactional systems." The loss of a person, or of some function from a system, occasions a sense of loss and grief. A person who at work was the prankster or the life of the party will be missed when she or he leaves. This loss will be felt not only for the person, but because a function the person fulfilled is now empty. Family systems sometimes have a hard time coping with loss. One man writes,

> Driving home from dropping off my daughter at college for her first semester, I experienced a great feeling of loss that she had now left our family circle and *our family life would never be the same.* This was the first instance of one of our children reaching college age, and though intellectually I was prepared for this I found that emotionally I wasn't.

Almost any loss will be a mixture of more than one of the six types mentioned. There are other variations in loss. There is avoidable and unavoidable loss, temporary and permanent loss, actual and imagined loss, anticipated and unanticipated loss. There is leaving and being left.

Whatever the circumstances, we grieve all kinds of losses. As we learn to grieve, to recover, to heal, we have learned important lessons. We have learned something about how to face the loss by death of those we hold dear. We begin to be ready for that multi-dimensional permanent loss that will be our own death.

Stages of Dying—Lessons to Be Learned

Out of her conversations with many people, Elizabeth Kubler-Ross drew some conclusions about the process of dying. She felt she discovered that terminally ill persons go through five stages of dying. As she recognized, not all persons experience all stages. Further, a person does not necessarily leave one stage to go on to the others. A person may vacillate between the stages at times. However, she contended, the map offers insights for healthily dealing with the fact and process of one's dying.

These, then, are the five stages of dying as Kubler-Ross observed them:

1. *Denial.* "No, not me." As a first response to news of coming death, denial is important and a very common step, as it helps cushion the impact of the dread news.

2. *Rage and anger.* "Why me?" The patient is likely to be most resentful that he or she will die while others remain healthy and alive. The anger may be general and vague, or it may be directed at God, physician and hospital staff, the family, or all of them.

3. *Bargaining.* "Yes, me, but . . ." The patient begins to accept the fact of his or her death but bargains for more time.

4. *Depression.* "Yes, me." Here there are two types of depression: reactive and preparatory. The person experiencing reactive depression mourns past losses, tasks not accomplished, wrongs committed. Then the person moves on to a state of preparatory grief as he or she prepares for the loss of all living experience, of all present objects, of life itself. During this stage a person may withdraw from other people, having finished his or her business with them. However, those standing by should not abandon the patient. They should, however, be understanding if the patient needs their presence less.

5. *Acceptance.* "My time is very close, and it's all right."[8]

In chart form, the road map of the stages of dying looks like this.[9]

The Stages of Dying Road Map[10]

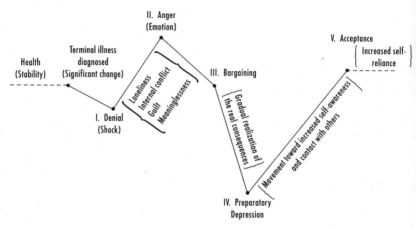

All of us are indebted to Kubler-Ross for opening up the subject of dying with such compassion and concern. She has gone on to do much more reflection on the subject of death and dying, including persons dying of AIDS. While she has recognized some variations in these stages, they have been repeatedly mentioned in literature on death and dying. At the same time, we need to realize that people's experiences are not nearly as linear as it might appear on a chart. Further, her conceptual framework is not the only one.

There are others who have looked at the process that dying persons experience and find something else. Edwin Shneidman described the dying process not by stage theory, but as a flow of negative and positive feelings. He compares this to the movement of bees in a hive. There is alternation of denial and fear, of rage and surrender, of hope and despair.

In his story *The Death of Ivan Ilych*, Leo Tolstoy has looked at his experience and that of others. The picture he offered was of this alternate flow of feelings. He describes the way a person might shift back and forth between denial, anger, and depression. The person may alternate between hope and despair. In Tolstoy's telling, this person finally came to acceptance at the very end of his struggle.

Each of these suggest that one's process in coping with one's own and others' finitude is varied and unique. One should not have a preset plan imposed on one in such sensitive matters. However, these writers do give clues that one *can* be healthy or unhealthy in the way one responds to one's own or another's coming death.

M. Scott Peck looks favorably on Kubler-Ross's stage theory of dying. However, he points out that many people have not reached the stage of acceptance at their death. He suggests that the reason is that it is too painful for them to reach that point. They may experience much agony in the anger, or bargaining, or particularly in the depression stage. The anguish may be so great that they may retreat back to denial. He sees this as regrettable, for acceptance is such a beautiful stage. He has experienced persons who have reached it as having such a mystical, transcendent quality. It is almost as if they have already died and are resurrected to a new realm. He hopes that more people find the help they need to do their work on their anger, or their depression. In such ways, they increase their chances of dying whole.[11]

This understanding of the thought processes of dying patients is important for us midlife people. They offer some insight for the midlifer as he or she makes the pilgrimage through life to death. Note that these five stages start with denial—the basic attitude toward death in our society. To be sure, modest change is occurring. There are now death and dying courses, support groups for grieving folks, funeral and memorial societies, and hospices. However, for the most part society denies that death exists. So do funeral homes, at least in some ways. So do most persons in their childhood, youth, and young adult years.

Then comes one of the crises of midlife. Changing bodies, death of parents, and possible other events make it less possible to deny death as a personal future event. (Up to this point I have been able to accept that you will one day die, but not that I will.) The certainty of one's own death begins to dawn.

Because death still seems fairly remote, we midlifers probably jumble together Kubler-Ross's stages of anger, bargaining, and depression. All of these may sneak up on us at times in our middle years. Occasionally we will experience unexpected anger, or, perhaps, deep depression. If we look behind these feelings, we probably will come face to face with the shortness of our life. Ignoring and denying this affords no release. Living with this dilemma in the presence of others who are in the same state can be helpful.

Repeatedly, the midlifer experiences limited time, frustration of dreams, and surgery, illness, or other reminders from one's body. We discover that one lifetime will not be long enough to do all the things we had hoped to do.

The midlifer comes to the conclusion not that "time is up," but rather that "time is limited." Out of this awareness can come the wisest stewardship of time. It might be well to imagine oneself terminally ill and ask, "If I were dying, what would be the relationships I would most savor, the tasks in which I would take most pride, the beliefs and causes that I would want to perpetuate?" Then one can resolve to come to death with as little depression over unlived life as possible.

Sometime, usually near the end of middle-age years, a person can move on to the stage of acceptance: "I want to live as long and as well as possible, but somehow, death is going to be all right." When, during midlife, a person has gone beyond the all-too-common death denial of our society and achieved a measure of acceptance, then one can be assured that he or she will live more fully and much more calmly face the final act of dying.

OUR RANGE OF CHOICES ABOUT DYING

When I deny my dying, I also deny myself the privilege of making intelligent choices concerning the subject of my death. Only when I have reached enough of a state of acceptance that my death is discussable, does a wide range of choices become possible.

I cannot decide whether or not I will die. However, I can decide many things, including the following.

To maintain and improve relationships in the knowledge that death will one day interrupt them. A few years ago, I was subject to a death threat. It came on a wintry morning. I discovered a truth I had once read somewhere: "When one knows one is to be hanged in a fortnight, it clears the mind wonderfully!" The very first thing that came to mind was my relationship with one particular family member. The relationship was not that bad, but it had some unresolved matters. Neither of us would have wanted that relationship to be where it was at the time of one of our deaths. One of the first things I chose to do was to take steps to resolve our differences.

To extend my life as long as reasonably possible. I can form good health habits as described in chapter 2, take the health exams fitting for my age and gender, and choose an attitude that is life-affirming and life-extending.

Not to extend my life beyond what is reasonably possible. This has become a hot issue in the 1990s. Dr. Jack Kevorkian invented and used a "death machine." In this manner, he assisted persons who had decided that they would rather die than go through the final stages of an illness. This action has been widely publicized, debated, and investigated. Many ethicists are wondering if there is another way to be responsive to the pain-ridden terminally ill. Derek Humphry's book *Final Exit: The Practicalities of Self-Deliverance and Assisted Suicide for the Dying* was highlighted in a *Wall Street Journal* article and became a nationwide best-seller. In this book, Humphry reflects on his own earlier writings and on the contribution of Dr. Kevorkian. Then he contends, "The taboo on suicide for reasons of health has been broken since 1980. . . . While it may need to be addressed in terms of social and health care policy, it does not deserve spontaneous condemnation."[12]

Humphry notes that the "euthanasia option" occurs in two ways. There is the passive option—disconnecting life-support equipment without which one cannot live. With appropriate advance steps (Living Will and/or Durable Power of Attorney, about which we will speak shortly) this may be done legally. There is also the active option—taking intentional steps to end one's life.

Though he believes in the rightness of this decision for some people, he warns that assisting in suicide is still a felony. Humphry points out that approximately half of all people in Western society die connected to life-support equipment. So the passive option may be viable for that half. For the other half, he insists, options ought to be available as well.[13] He then goes on to discuss steps in making such a decision, matters to deal with before dying, and lethal dosages of drugs that can kill a person.

Humphry brings a public debate and discussion that needs to be faced. The revolution of health care technology brings with it some hard questions. Each person and each family will need to reach decisions on these matters. Personally, I would be willing to administer or receive "passive euthanasia" if my condition were hopeless and the machines were simply extending dying. I could not, in all good conscience, enter into the active euthanasia option of which he speaks.

If people share the viewpoint that passive euthanasia may be an acceptable option, they need to take two steps. One is to sign a "living will" and have it witnessed. Then copies of it should be placed with one's physician and others who might have a part in health decisions. Copies of living wills are available from hospices and physicians. While one may make qualifications on it, this document basically says that one does not wish to be connected to life-support equipment if one is hopelessly and terminally ill. It also gives permission to disconnect such systems. Persons may name what life support they want and what they do not want and the conditions they would want this applied. A living will only comes into effect if the person who made it is unconscious or lacks the capability to make the decision at the moment of treatment. Helpful as this document may be, in many situations it is not legally binding. Rather, it may be a valuable aid to those who must make such decisions.

A more powerful document is the Durable Power of Attorney for Health Care. With this, one assigns to someone else the power to make health care decisions when the signer is unable to make them. This document is legally enforceable, while the living will, quite probably, is not.

There is another point at which people will have occasion to think about these decisions. With the passage of the "Patient Self-Determination Act," all federally funded hospitals in the United States are required to advise patients of their right to make out living wills and express their will about such matters.

More and more, when a person enters a hospital, that person will be asked about "advance directives." That is, what is the patient's wish about being resuscitated if her or his heart stops? What is the patient's desire regarding "extraordinary means" if the patient is brain dead or in a permanently vegetative state? Much of the money expended on health care goes to extend low-quality life in the last months of living. Therefore, a family may want to discuss these matters and support one another in decisions.

As we mentioned, probably one will have to explore these concerns with one's aged parents or grandparents before facing them for oneself. It will be helpful to discuss these matters before they occur. However, it may be extremely difficult to do so.

With today's health care technology, such questions are virtually inescapable. Fortunate is the family that has empowered itself with advance discussions and decisions. It will be able to face those inevitable decisions with more strength and peace.

To let go with love those persons who are terminally ill and dying. Beyond the technical steps described in the previous point, dying persons may feel they are letting people down if they die. And so they may hang on, with a low-quality, painful life. Bernie Siegel urges folks at this point to give the dying person permission to go. Love, support, and grief should be shared. But they should also share the affirmation that though they will miss their loved one, they will be OK.[14]

I was able to do this with my mom, a few months before she died. I had been called because a crisis had come and caregivers thought death might be near. That particular crisis had passed, but she was weakened and very uncomfortable. I told her, "Mom, as active as you have always been, I'm sure this confinement is tough. I'm proud of the way you have handled it. I know that life is more and more difficult for you. If the time comes that you want to let go, I will understand. I love you and will miss you. But you have prepared us well. We will be OK." She thanked me. While she wasn't quite ready to go, she said, she thought that time might be close. And, she would remember what I said. While my family has not always been one to say the things that need to be said, we did get through this with each other. That conversation still comforts me even though when death was much closer, Mom's communication about it was nonverbal.

To enter freely and openly into grieving for loved ones who have died. Psychologists have noted three major stages of grieving. The first is *impact*. This is a period of catastrophe when the blow of death is first absorbed. This may be a time of numbness. It may last for days or months.

The second stage, *recoil*, is when shock and numbness is replaced by a stark knowledge that the death is real and the person is permanently gone. This may last for days, months, or years.

With healthy grieving, there comes a third stage, *recovery*. Marks of this stage are acceptance, willingness to say goodbye, willingness to grant the dead person a place in history and to get on with living.[15]

There are many moods and emotions that often go with grieving. Among these are numbness; loneliness, emptiness, and isolation; fear and anxiety; guilt and shame; anger; sadness and despair; and somatization (that is, symptoms in the body such as tightness in the throat, sighing, lack of muscular power, etc.).[16]

Having said all this, grief is quite an individual experience. There is no way to predict its course, what will stir it, or what form it will take.

About a month after Mom died, I stopped in a card shop to buy a wedding anniversary card for friends. Unconsciously, I moved over an aisle, since the Mother's Day cards were out. I browsed for a few minutes before it hit me. I couldn't send her one this year. Reminders that stir grief will happen again and again, mostly from unexpected quarters. An object, a song, a smell, almost anything can strike a blow on the grief wound, revealing how far from healed it is.

I discovered what many others have known: that grief is a braid with several strands. While working on the memories project I described, some surprising feelings surfaced. There was a tremendous amount of sadness over how little I knew about my dad and how much I missed his companionship, partnership in the same profession, and his wisdom. This surprised me because my dad had been dead over forty years. I thought I was over that. I realized that Mom, my sister, and I had tried hard to fill that gap for each other. With Mom gone, the gap reappeared.

Though painful, grief is not to be avoided. Only when we grieve fully can we remember joyfully. Only when we accept the pain can we experience the bright thoughts. Tears and laughter are kindred expressions.

Quite frequently, in going through my daily work I will come upon something that reminds me of my pal Lee. I almost pick up the phone to call him. The memory might be of an experience we shared, some shenanigan we pulled off, a joke we enjoyed together. I find myself smiling and chuckling with tears in my eyes and a lump in my throat. But that's OK. The pain I still often feel is not too great a price to pay for those precious relationships with my mother and with Lee. Allowing the grief to flow to healing colors my life richly.

What to do with my body after I die. Recently, Joshua Elliott, a delightful, energetic six-year-old boy in my congregation, suddenly contracted meningitis and was found to be brain dead. In the midst of this tragedy, his parents requested donation of any organs that would be useful to others. His right kidney went to a fifteen-year-old boy in Iowa, and his left kidney to a forty-seven-year-old woman in California, the mother of a nineteen-year-old. His liver went to an eight-year-old girl in California, and his heart valves (which can be preserved longer) were available for heart surgery as needed.

This act of courageous compassion by these grieving parents touched me deeply. On the day I heard of it, I did something I had long delayed—I signed the statement on the back of my driver's license ("I hereby make an anatomical gift effective upon my death") and had my signature witnessed.

Each of us may want to make some decisions about the use of our body after we die.

- Would I like to make available usable organs or tissues from my body for the living?
- Would I like to will my body for medical research?
- How do I want my body treated for funeral and burial purposes? Do I desire cremation? A simple, inexpensive burial? If so, I may want to do "pre-planning" with a funeral director or a funeral and memorial society. One may want to do this for members of one's family as well. It can prevent emotional overspending at the stressful time of death.

How I want my faith and values expressed in the rituals after I die. As a pastor I keep a file of requests that people have made, formally or informally, about their desires for their funeral or memorial service. You may have scriptures, readings, music, statements of faith that express the meaning of your life. You may want these used as a witness at the time of your death.

To whom and for what purposes I want any remaining assets to be left. If I have not expressed myself, the state will provide for this in a logical manner, but one that may not fit my concerns. I may want to make specific provision for persons I love, for beliefs I hold high, for causes and organizations I treasure. If that is my desire, I need to do so specifically. I may want to elect life insurance (which is actually death insurance) to make provision for persons or causes important to me.

The Ways We Seek and Claim Immortality

The proper use of a life is to invest it in something that will outlast it. One needs to know that it mattered that she or he lived. If one cannot be around consciously participating in the events or future generations, can he or she at least know that in some way he or she endures?

Robert Lifton and Eric Olson address this question with their concept of "symbolic immortality." They suggest that one experiences a sense of immortality in five "modes" or categories. (These modes may be more meaningful in some cultures than in others.)

The first mode is *"biological* immortality," meaning that one lives on through sons and daughters and their sons and daughters.

Second is the mode of *"works,"* or the *"creative"* mode. "One may feel a sense of immortality . . . through teaching, art-making, repairing, construction, writing, healing, inventing, or through lasting influences of any kind on other human beings—influences that one feels can enter into a general human flow beyond the self."[17]

Third, the *"theological"* mode of immortality is that set of beliefs that affirms the person's place in the eternal plans of God.

The fourth mode is immortality achieved through *"continuity with nature."* "You are dust, and to dust you shall return" (Gen. 3:19) is not only an Old Testament warning against pride. It is also the affirmation of affinity with nature that endures beyond the person, but of which the person is a part. Whatever happens to human beings, trees, mountains, rivers, and seas endure. We sense this and return to nature for spiritual refreshment and revitalization.

A fifth mode of immortality is *"experiential transcendence"*; that is, going beyond the limits and confines of ordinary daily life in some experience of ecstasy. This might be found in a religious encounter, but it may also be found in "music, dance, battle, athletics, mechanical flight, contemplation of the past, artistic or intellectual creation, sexual love, childbirth, comradeship, and the feeling of working together with others in common cause."[18]

Therefore, say Lifton and Olson, five modes are available to us to participate in that which endures. Within these modes we are granted symbolic immortality.

What Dying May Teach Us

If we have heeded the counsel in the preceding pages, we may be growing in our living with dying. We may have begun to reorder our priorities for wise use of this precious limited life we have. We may reach a state when we are assured that we partake in that which will endure. We begin to understand that death is part of living. We progress on to a preliminary participation in the last stage of attitudes toward dying—acceptance. Our search at midlife is ultimately a spiritual one.

At this point we may be ready to hear information from yet another quarter. Those who are facing death or have been near death have much to teach us. They tell us that rather than something to be feared, death can be something beautiful in itself. And it can be the occasion for amazing growth.

Here is one example. Murray L. Trelease, in recalling his experience among Native Americans in Seattle, writes:

> I remember a nineteen year old boy dying of leukemia who in two weeks' time grew from a rather irresponsible brat to a loving, understanding counselor who led his family through the shattering experience of his dying. When he first learned he was dying he could think of nothing but rejection and resentment. But a short time later he discovered that he had a long agenda of things he wanted to know and understand. There were people to see, old sores to heal, his family to help and comfort; he was still thinking of more things to accomplish when he died suddenly . . . the sentence of death . . . may mark the beginning of the greatest growth of a lifetime in understanding, love, and faith.[19]

Consider a viewpoint from a much different quarter. Famed psychologist Abraham Maslow suffered a life-threatening heart attack. When he was recovering, he spoke of his "post-mortem life," and wrote these words:

> The confrontation with death—and the reprieve from it—makes everything look so precious, so sacred, so beautiful, that I feel more strongly than ever the impulse to love it, to embrace it, and

to let myself be overwhelmed by it. . . . Death, and its ever present
possibility makes love, passionate love, more possible. I wonder if
we could love passionately, if ecstasy would be possible at all, if we
knew we'd never die.[20]

Let us consider one more witness, this from Raymond A.
Moody Jr., who investigated over 150 cases of people who had
near-death experiences, or had been pronounced clinically dead
and then had been resuscitated. Moody discovered a good bit of
variety in what they recalled, but there were some common
themes as well.

He describes the most incredible common element that these
persons experienced as an encounter with a very bright light. Often this light begins very dimly, but quickly becomes brighter until it reaches an unearthly brilliance. All the persons Moody
interviewed seemed to be sure that this light was a personal being,
a being of light, with a very definite personality. They experienced
a love and warmth emanating from this being. The dying person
sensed that she or he was completely surrounded by it, taken up in
it, at peace with it, and accepted. The light was an irresistible mag-
netic attraction. The person was drawn to it.

Moody summarized what these persons told him they had
learned from their close encounters with death:

> There is a remarkable agreement in the 'lessons,' as it were, which
> have been brought back from these close encounters with death.
> Almost everyone has stressed the importance in this life of trying
> to cultivate love for others, a love of unique and profound kind. . . .
> In addition, many others have emphasized the importance of seek-
> ing knowledge. During their experiences, it was intimated to them
> that the acquisition of knowledge continues even in the after-
> life. . . . Their vision left them with new goals, new moral princi-
> ples, and a renewed determination to try to live in accordance with
> them.[21]

The witness of these persons seems to be that death has a
twofold dimension. For one thing, it is a closed door. Its message

to us is to learn, serve, relate, love in the limited time we have. But death also is an open door, a vista to new mysteries and majesties that we have not yet discovered.

Faith and Finitude

What is the connection between the Christian faith and our finitude? Several interrelationships readily come to mind.

First, there is the discovery of Dr. Kubler-Ross that while nominal or external religion is no help at all to dying people (and is sometimes a hindrance), "intensely religious people accept death more easily than others . . . if they are authentic and have internalized their faith. The significant variable is . . . how truly and genuinely you believe. Truly religious people with a deep abiding relationship with God have found it much easier to face death with equanimity."[22]

Second, however, there is a caution we must consider. I fear that often people of faith have participated in that death denial that is so pervasive in our culture. What I mean is that we speak so glibly of immortality, heaven, life after death, resurrection, etc., that we ignore and deny the reality of death. Whatever the Christian faith promises, it does not promise that Christians escape dying. An individual still must come to grips with his or her own dying and must face one's own death. When someone he or she cares about dies first, the Christian is not spared any of the loneliness, agony, or grief work that accompanies such a loss.

Therefore, the Christian must be careful not to overclaim or underclaim what the Christian faith may provide in the face of death. One overclaims when one insists that our faith makes dying something one does easily, with eager anticipation. (Many Christian songs about dying and heaven fall into just this error.) But one should not underclaim what the Christian faith offers in this regard either. Both the New Testament and contemporary believers show us that our faith helps us face death openly with trust and hope. In short, what faith offers is death transformation, not death denial. I will discuss this further in a moment.

Third, Jesus, the central figure of our faith, lived among us, suffered, and died. As I read those detailed accounts in the Gospels, I detect that he went through stages of dying similar to those Kubler-Ross described. For example, is there not possible bargaining, anger, and depression in the words "If it is possible, let this cup pass from me" (Matt. 26:39); "My God, my God, why have you forsaken me?" (Matt. 27:46); "It is finished" (John 19:30)? Then in his final moments, is there not the mood of acceptance: "Father, into your hands I commit my spirit!" (Luke 23:46)? Further, Hebrews 5:7 reminds us, "In the days of his flesh, Jesus offered up prayers and supplications, with loud cries and tears, to the one who was able to save him from death."

My personal belief is strengthened by this discovery. I discover that my God entered so fully into my humanity through Jesus that Jesus died with similar emotions and personal processes to those I must face. Jesus models for me how to die and offers me knowledgeable companionship. This helps me as I face the fact of my own death and the deaths of those I love.

By entering into the process of dying with and for us, Jesus conquered sin and death. The victory established through his death means that death is transformed. We die from a different perspective than we would have without him (1 Cor. 15:57).

Fourth, as I seek the "symbolic immortality" of which Lifton speaks, I find the consolations of the Christian faith at every point:

Biological immortality. In the very process of begetting children I have been drawn up into partnership with God and have become creator with God. The Old Testament affirms that children are a means to immortality in that one's influence and name are perpetuated.

"Works," or "creative," immortality. Recall the final verse of Psalm 90, that great poem on God's eternity and our mortality.

Let the favor of our God be upon us, and prosper for us the work of our hands—O prosper the work of our hands. (Ps. 90:17)

The psalmist trustfully asks God to take the things he had done, accept them, and "establish them," make them endure.

Immortality through continuity with nature. Our faith affirms this channel as well. A psalmist writes,

> I lift up my eyes to the hills—from where will my help come? My help comes from [God], who made heaven and earth. (Ps. 121:1–2)

Again and again, Bible writers with eyes of faith see God's creation and its renewal as a sign of hope for us human beings. Burial services remind us that we come from earth and return to earth and are part of the new life the earth will bring forth.

Immortality through "experiential transcendence." That is, experiences of ecstasy wherever they occur. The Bible tells us that our experiences of fellowship with God, those moments of ecstasy, are the preview sample of the glory we will share. Jesus tells us, "And this is eternal life, that they know you, the only true God, and Jesus Christ whom you have sent" (John 17:3). Since we affirm a God who created all, we have no problem accepting the idea that any moment of ecstasy in music, art, contemplation, comradeship, etc., is indeed a gift of God symbolizing that which meaningfully endures.

While these four of Lifton's and Olson's "modes" of "symbolic immortality" are not ignored in biblical faith, we must pause for a caution. None of these four is distinctively Christian. Furthermore, neither "biological immortality" nor "works or creative immortality" is available to all. Further still, dependence on these four modes would be idolatry, as they are modes that "trust" in blood lines (children), creative works (works of righteousness), nature worship, or the self. These modes do have important meanings, but these meanings must be peripheral for the Christian, never central. This brings us to the central mode for the Christian.

Theological immortality. Our Christian faith offers a theological view of death transformed, not death denied. Jesus' resurrection was a new and powerful divine event in the world. God acted upon that death to confirm Jesus' costly sacrifice, to awaken us to Jesus' continued power and influence in the world, and to assure us that "whether we live or whether we die, we are [God's]" (Rom. 14:8).

When we discover how gently our Christian faith leads us into the acceptance of death with faith and hope, we may gain a deeper trust both about the deaths of those we love and the death of each of us. We let death teach us the valuable growth lessons it has for us. In this way we are led to cherish each other, the joyous moments granted us, and life itself. Ever more fully we are led to join with that affirmation Thornton Wilder made at the end of his novel *The Bridge of San Luis Rey*:

> And we ourselves shall be loved for a while and forgotten. But the love will have been enough; all those impulses of love return to the love that made them. Even memory is not necessary for love. There is a land of the living and a land of the dead, and the bridge is love, the only survival, the only meaning.[23]

For Personal or Group Reflection and Discussion

1. What persons have modeled calm acceptance of death (in self or others) for you? What did you discover from them?

2. In the section on choices about dying, which choices have you already made? With which are you wrestling? Which are you avoiding? Of the decisions you have made, have you discussed them with the persons who need to know?

3. How do you feel about the discussion of passive and active euthanasia? Can you see yourself agreeing to either measure? Why or why not?

4. Personally or as a group, you might want to invite a physician or other health care professional to discuss Living Wills, Durable Power of Attorney for Health Care, and advance directives.

5. What affirmations of the Christian faith speak to you most powerfully as you consider the deaths of those you love and your own death? What unresolved questions do you have?

Resources

Bianchi, Eugene C. *Aging as a Spiritual Journey*. New York: Crossroad, 1982, 1989.

Conway, Jim. *Men in Mid-Life Crisis*. Elgin, Ill: David C. Cook, 1972, 1982.

Grief Education Institute—Board of Trustees. *Bereavement Support Groups: Leadership Manual*. Denver: Grief Education Institute, 1987.

Humphry, Derek. *Final Exit: The Practicalities of Self-Deliverance and Assisted Suicide for the Dying*. Eugene, Oreg.: The Hemlock Society, 1991.

Kubler-Ross, Elizabeth. *Death: The Final Stage of Growth*. Englewood Cliffs, N.J.: Prentice-Hall, 1975.

———. *On Death and Dying*. New York: Macmillan, 1969.

Lifton, Robert Jay, and Eric Olson. *Living and Dying*. New York: Praeger, 1974.

Loewinsohn, Ruth Jean. *Survival Handbook for Widows*. Chicago: Follett Publishing, 1979.

Mitchell, Kenneth R., and Herbert Anderson. *All Our Losses, All Our Griefs*. Philadelphia: Westminster Press, 1983.

Moody, Raymond A., Jr. *Life after Life*. New York: Bantam Books, 1973, 1976.

Peck, M. Scott. *Further Along the Road Less Traveled: The Unending Journey toward Spiritual Growth*. New York: Simon and Schuster, 1993.

Siegel, Bernie S. *Love, Medicine, and Miracles*. New York: Harper and Row, 1986.

Worden, J. William, and William Proctor. *Personal Death Awareness*. Englewood Cliffs, N.J.: Prentice-Hall, 1976.

9

Exploring Myself and My Faith

L ET'S PAUSE A MOMENT and reflect on our process thus far in this book. In chapter 1 we explored an overview of the life journey and midlife in particular. We discovered that life gives us a wide-ranging agenda on which to work in the middle years! There are outer and inner tasks. From there we went on to explore a number of those outer tasks in detail. Our next step is to consider inward work we have to do.

L. Patrick Carroll and Katherine Marie Dyckman note that at midlife a pervasive issue is the loss of youth. Further, a basic faith issue we must deal with is our sense of brokenness. And a central psychological issue is the demise of our myth about ourselves. They continue:

> We are invited in the middle of the stream of life to deal with the unfinished business of the past, to cope with the physical changes that assail us. We are aware as never before of issues of affectivity, intimacy, sexuality that need to be settled. We are equally aware of a growing sense of our mortality —we and all whom we love will die, in fact are dying. We wonder how to sustain faith when God seems absent or perhaps is no longer imaged as benign. . . . We wonder who we are and what we are worth. And all of this goes on more or less at the same moment.[1]

In other words, in midlife God gets our attention, and invites us to a new self-understanding. To respond to this invitation, we need a many-faceted inner growth. As we noted, this inner growth begins with an acceptance of death as a part of life. There is a resulting freedom to live one's limited days with freedom and intentionality.

Here are some of the aspects of that further inner growth as I discern them.

I Search for a Clearer Self-Understanding

This search for a clearly understood self-concept has been going on over a lifetime. The two-year-old's self-definition by means of the word "no" . . . the child's and youth's frequent concern, "What do my friends think of me?" . . . the late adolescent's experimentation, rebellion, and (perhaps temporary) rejection of family values . . . the later consideration, "Is it OK to say yes to some of those values?" . . . all of this and more has contributed to a person's self-understanding.

Still, there is much truth in Janice Brewi and Anne Brennan's comment, "Whereas accommodation was the key word for the tasks of the first half of life, individuation is the key word for the second half of life." This individuation may be filled in with such terms as "inwardness . . . self-realization, integration, reconciliation, coming to self-hood."[2]

The expectations for the development of a person in childhood, youth, and young adult years is quite clearly described. There are expectations for each of the years 3, 6, 9, 16, 18, 21, and 30. There are messages from a wide variety of sources about what one should do and what one should become. Parents, teachers, experts, siblings, friends, employers, mentors all give input. Brewi and Brennan note,

> The ego development of the child and youth, hopefully, is a genuine development, true to the personality; yet we must realize it is also a development of accommodation. . . . The child responds to fit into the expectations of society.[3]

At midlife, each of us needs to become our own parent, teacher, friend, and mentor. We come to understand that the life stages and tasks we have undergone are necessary, but they are only provisional and preliminary stages to full human development. We are faced with the task of looking within to claim a unique self. The directions come not from the outside but from within. There may be recognition of personal attributes dimly known or unknown. These may be gifts that need to be recognized and celebrated. There may be reaffirmation of aspects of self that others have not encouraged. There may be spiritual longings and hungers that for years have been dulled by busyness and outward demands. Or they may never before have been recognized.

A person may also encounter some unpleasant things in this look within. There may be a sense of unlived life, or the feeling that part of one's life has been a lie. One may discover misdirection and inappropriate courses in the past. There may be a growing awareness that we are not the person we thought we were. It is not surprising that frequently pain and depression go with this inner journey.

This intense look within—once or many times in the middle years—is an entirely normal and needed effort. However, it is little understood and not greatly encouraged in our society. Therefore intentionality, courage, and energy are needed to undertake it.

Why would anyone undertake any exploration that has so much discomfort in it? Carl Jung, who noted the terrain of midlife experience, suggests two reasons for this undertaking. On the one hand, Jung contended that those who refuse to face these hard questions and try to live the second half of life by the same principles as the first were doomed to be "hypochondriacs, niggards, doctrinaires, applauders of the past or eternal adolescents—all lamentable substitutes for the illumination of the self."[4]

Not only is there a disappointment to be avoided, there is a treasure to be gained. This treasure is the full flowering of one's personality, a personal renaissance, a rebirth. William Johnston writes:

I believe that in this psychological turmoil [of midlife self-examination] grace is working gently, if painfully, in the unconscious inviting . . . our true selves, to emerge from the womb into fullness of life. Quite often the whole process of middle age crisis is nothing less than a mystical experience of death and resurrection to a new life which is filled with true joy.[5]

We will return to the topic of possible new births in the next chapter.

There is a deeply theological/spiritual dimension to what we are describing. We will explore that dimension in more detail later in this chapter and in the next.

So far I have described this self-exploration in stark and sweeping terms. Quite probably many will discover that they have anticipated and embarked on much of this self-discovery and course correction earlier. They may feel that only modest changes and adjustments are necessary. That can be an affirming experience in itself.

Still, there will be times when one will need to be in vital touch with this inner journey in order to weather outside assaults on the person one understands oneself to be. I had just such an experience recently—in late midlife, after I thought I had worked through much of this. I was going through a time of grief and depression, and, truth be known, something of a slump in my personal and work life. As I lived with the extended effects of the double grief I described in the last chapter, I became more somber and withdrawn than usual. Even before that, there had been some discontent with my leadership at the church where I was pastor. In all this, from a variety of persons, there came suggestions that I should change myself in several basic ways—personality (more folksy and outgoing), theology (more conservative), style as a public speaker (more dynamic, entertaining, and funny).

Fear warned me, "Pay attention—you could get yourself fired." Inner strength somehow was able to say, "I'd rather be fired for being who I am than for being a clone of a person I don't even know."

There was personal freedom and power for me in that answer. Whatever the source of the challenge, whatever the time in life, this inner redirection is an important and powerful step for each person in the middle third of life. It may be one huge consideration or a series of smaller ones.

I Reexplore My Dreams and Vocation

It is hard to overestimate the importance of dreams in adult development. When we were young adults each of us formulated a dream for our life. This may include career, achievements, relationships, family, and more.

Evelyn Eaton Whitehead and James D. Whitehead have explored the midlife task of processing such dreams from a distinctively Christian perspective. They note the close correlation between Christian vocation and dreams. Vocation is God's call or invitation to "make something good and holy of our lives."[6] It is the lifelong task of every person to carry on a conversation with God about this, and to receive the clues, hints, guidance one is given about one's vocation. A part of this discovery may come through dreams about one's life.

There are close connections between the psychological notion of a life's dream and the Christian understanding of vocation. Both are our deepest and best hopes for our lives. Both arise out of the person's imagination. Christians may see dreams, therefore, as vehicles for God's revelation of one's vocation. At the same time, dreams may not necessarily be revelations from God. And if they are such at one point in life, they may not be at a later time.

Therefore the midlife years provide an opportunity to do some delicate examining of one's earlier dreams. We hope to discover what about our dreams are also God's dreams, and therefore part of our present and future vocation. This might be called reexamining our dreams, seeking reconciliation with our dreams, or purifying our expectations. There are several alternatives.

In one pattern, I may need to come to terms with how the dream has gone. The early dream may have been idealistic and grand. The way it has been lived was probably more realistic. I may need to undergo "de-illusionment"—not disillusionment. It may be to let go some of youth's necessary illusions. I can rejoice in what the dream has contributed to my person and achievements. I can mourn the parts that probably will not be achieved and can accept the dream's function in my life.

In yet another pattern, I may need to recognize the tyranny of the dream in my life. Perhaps one aspect of a dream has been pursued so that other important parts of the dream have been sacrificed. Reconciliation with this type of dream means release from its tyranny. I may need to recover parts of life that were ignored or denied. It may be I need to forgive myself for falling into an overemphasized, one-sided tyrannical dream.

Or I may be called to recover a dream that was deferred. There may be the discovery that an earlier dream has been lost. I may have been sidetracked or talked out of the dream, or I may have lost sight of it. Again I will need to forgive part of my past. This self-forgiveness is a necessary component in allowing the dream's energy and attractive power to come to the fore once more.

And again, I may need to recognize that a dream needs to be let go, to be allowed to die. It may have had importance for my life for a while, but no longer. Or it may have been one of those dreams that one can clearly now see was not part of God's dream for my life. What is needed is a clear break with such a dream.

At the same time I will need to be open to a new dream to take the place of the one surrendered. The end of one dream may be the beginning of another.[7]

There may be yet another challenge. What if my dream has been fulfilled in all of its essential aspects? Fulfilled dreams and reached goals give a person a remarkably short-lived satisfaction. Someone once wrote, "The gods mock us by denying us our dreams or by granting them." That seems rather cynical, but the question remains—what does one do after one's dream is substantially fulfilled? Perhaps the answer is—be open to another dream. God may call through that dream. History has many stories of persons who launch out on new ventures after fulfilling goals that others envy.

As we reconcile with our dreams, we are called to do this in harmony with dreams of our families and communities of faith. We are also to be in concert with God's dreams for humanity—the reign of God. The Whiteheads summarize:

> A Christian vocation may be described as a dream, God's dream for my life, developing in my imagination. Such a dream is gradually revealed to us in the various achievements and reversals of adult life. Since it is sometimes fragile, a personal vocation may be neglected and then wither. Or it may become compulsive and too well defended. Christian ministry always entails a fostering of dreams: clarifying and purifying our vocations, we come closer to imagining what God is about in our lives.[8]

In midlife, I reconsider my dreams and my vocation.

I Come to an Inner Recognition of Life's Complexities

Part of midlife inner growth is the discovery that some issues in life are much more complex, vague, and difficult than previously imagined. Dorothy Parker once put this very well in her poem "The Veteran."

> When I was young and bold and strong,
> Oh, right was right and wrong was wrong.
> My plume on high, my flag unfurled,
> I rode away to fight the world.
> "Come out you dogs, and fight!" said I
> And wept, there was but once to die.
> But I am old and good and bad
> Are woven in a crazy plaid.
> I sit and say, "The world is so
> And he is wise who lets it go.
> A battle lost, a battle won,
> The difference is small, my son."
> Inertia rides and riddles me!
> The which is called philosophy.[9]

In chapter 1 we noted Roger Gould's observation that in adulthood there is need to shed the childish assumption that "life is simple and controllable." In our middle years we have a variety of experiences and inward processing that near overwhelms us with how complicated it all is.

This discovery might have to do with society and social causes. Earlier beliefs might have included these:

- If a cause is just it will triumph.
- The right leader with a committed group of followers can bring about this change.
- If I am talented, committed, and capable, I will be recognized and justly rewarded for my talents and efforts.

This discovery might have to do with personal issues, such as:

- I can become whatever I want to be.
- I can overcome any limitations, faults, or habits within me that might hinder me.

Quite possibly, by the middle years we will have experienced some disappointments in both our social and personal domains. We may have embraced movements in which we believed passionately but that now have failed or faded. We may have discovered how difficult it is to bring about change. There may have been leaders in whom we passionately believed who were killed or had difficulty delivering on promises if they lived. We may have discovered that issues about which we had strong convictions have two sides. To our surprise, we can see both sides of an issue now, and may even have changed sides! It may cause us chagrin that we have raised children who oppose our viewpoints as strongly as we resisted our parents' viewpoints.

We may have discovered how capricious, unfair, and unpredictable the workplace can be. Along with this, there may be the awakening that we may achieve less than we had imagined. (Recall an earlier definition of the beginning of midlife: that time when a person realizes that he or she will never be president of the firm.)

As if all this were not enough, we discover that our own personal growth and transformation is more problematical than we had thought earlier. The apostle Paul once wrote, "I do not understand my own actions. For I do not do what I want, but I do the very thing I hate" (Rom. 7:15). We can understand and resonate with that frustrated desire. Sir James Barry once wrote to the effect that each of us is two diaries: one about the person we want to be; one about the person we are. Our humblest moment comes when we realize how great the difference between the two.

Our inner journey has to do with how we manage such social and personal mysteries. We need to make our peace with complications such as complexity, ambiguity, and paradox. Complexity is the awareness of a multitude of factors to consider, with the acknowledgment that we probably never get all the factors in their proper relation to each other. Ambiguity is the awareness that there are aspects of an issue that cannot be known, perhaps not now, perhaps never. Paradox includes the acknowledgment that truth might be held in two seemingly opposite statements, which are held in tension with each other as the deeper truth is sought.

If we do not develop a way to engage these mysteries, we may lapse into cynicism, apathy, or indecisiveness. Russell Lynes once observed, "Cynicism is the intellectual cripple's substitute for intelligence." However, it is also a real temptation for persons lacking any other way to deal with life's frustrations and disappointments.

With a healthy, solemn respect for our own and society's mysteries, complexities, ambiguities, and paradoxes, we do not let go. Rather we seek a rekindled, though humbled, passion for those commitments that still summon us, both personal and societal.

I Look for Resources to Help Me Cope and Be Strong

"Life is difficult," said M. Scott Peck at the beginning of his bestselling book, *The Road Less Traveled*.[10] In this era of life, we discover how true that is.

Midlife—in and of itself—contains strain and struggle for those who go through it. The inner tasks we have already described:

plus being the middle generation with needs coming
   from both directions,
plus job and career pressures,
with some health concerns,
and with awareness of one's mortality,

is quite enough for the human psyche.

However, persons in the early and middle midlife years have yet other emotional burdens to bear. For one thing, there is an awareness for many people that they have not achieved as much by this point in their lives as their parents did (at least economically). Rather, downward mobility, or running hard to keep even with real income, is more the pattern.

Then, too, there seems to be a good bit of loneliness in these years. A large percentage of people have never married. Many married couples don't succeed in staying together. Some who divorce enter a remarriage with a blended-family situation that may be marked by a great deal of uncertainty about belonging and acceptance. It is estimated that one in three Americans suffer from loneliness. John Roschen observes, "At the heart of loneliness is estrangement from the caring of others that leads one to question one's own meaning.... Learning to encounter loneliness and the accompanying sadness is an essential part of midlife's faith-work."[11]

A kindred feeling is that of rootlessness. I may have rejected a good bit of the traditions of my childhood. While the search and the rebelling may have been exhilarating and needed, new questions need to be asked. In what values, teachings, traditions, faith do I trust? Where and how can I be grounded?

For these reasons or others there is a marked increase in depression in the baby boom generation. Estimates are that this generation experiences depression at three to ten times the rate of their parents. In this connection, there has also been a 300 percent increase in suicide in the last three decades. These and other indicators point out that the younger adult generation is having a more difficult adjustment to midlife than did their parents or grandparents.[12]

Each of us will need to find the resources not only to cope but to grow from such struggles. Personally, my resources will at least include the following: a good psychotherapist with whom I have established trust and whom I can call on when needed; print resources such as this one and those I am reporting, plus use of other media; a disciplined time for devotional practice, silence, listening to myself, listening for my God. Yet another resource is the admission that I cannot make it on my own, that I need all the others of whom I have spoken.

I Become Intentional about Relationships, Friendships, Groups

There is another richly helpful resource to assist me in dealing with the stress, loneliness, rootlessness, and depression of which I just spoke. That resource is other persons who are on the same journey. I need relationships with persons of both sexes, open and honest friendships, support groups.

This may mean that I reestablish ties with those to whom I was close in years past. Perhaps we can pick up on the trust we felt back in childhood, high school, college, military service, or whatever. Or it may mean that I inquire of present friends if they want to go to a deeper level of honesty, vulnerability, and support with each other. Or I may need to reach out and intentionally "court" some new friends. There may be persons with whom I have shared a brief experience that gave a clue that we could find some enriching wavelengths on which to share. I may choose to go to such persons and propose a deeper level of friendship.

One of the powerful movements in America is the small group movement. Quite likely this movement has grown in response to the loss of security in families, neighborhoods, and workplaces. With the loss of some of those characteristics of a good society, alternative forms need to be invented. Persons are discovering a new/old form—a support group of persons who gather together regularly and covenant honesty, confidentiality, a growing trust and sharing with each other. If I have not yet found such a group,

I may want to reach out to find one or create one. Perhaps I should find some friends with whom to discuss this book.

I Seek a Road Map of My Faith Journey

Two persons were discussing how they weathered some storms of change that occurred in midlife. Said one, "My faith was the one firm foundation on which I could depend with all the uncertainties I was experiencing." The other responded, "My faith was one of the things that was changing most of all. That was the most uncomfortable of all the fluctuations in my middle years."

Bidden or unbidden, we may experience faith changes through the middle third of life. These variations may be in the way we think about and process our beliefs, or in the content of our beliefs. In the next chapter we will talk about the content—for now, let's look the framework from which we do our faithing.

Over the last fifteen or twenty years, scholars have been exploring how faith develops or changes in a person. They suggest that "faith is a verb."[13] A verb is a word of action. In a sentence the verb "indicates movement, activity, direction, purpose. There is a dynamic quality about a verb. A verb indicates that *something is happening*."[14]

Each person will have one's own way of responding to the doctrines, beliefs, teachings of one's religious faith. I sort these out, recognizing what speaks most meaningfully and deeply to me. I walk through life with them, and sometimes discover that some teachings fade and others come into clearer focus. Kenneth Stokes suggests:

> Faith is always in process. . . . "Faith is a verb" suggests new dimensions with tremendous potential for all of us. . . . *My* faith is a unique blend of *my* background and *my* religious experience plus *my* development of body, mind, personality, social setting, and 1001 other dimensions of *my* being that makes *me* unique and different from everybody else. Ultimately *my* faith must be owned by *me*![15]

This does not deny the importance of religious teachings. Creeds and doctrines offer the starting point. Each person must work through what those mean and how they operate in the individual life. This is necessary to have a dynamic faith that one "owns." In such a way, a person's faith development proceeds. A number of persons have studied and reflected on this process. Let's take a look at a few.

JOHN WESTERHOFF
Styles of Faith

John Westerhoff compares this process to the growth of a tree. At any point in its life, a tree is whole and complete. However, it does add rings of growth as it ages and matures. Westerhoff suggests that there are at least four "rings" or styles of faithing.

The earliest style is "experienced faith." During preschool and early childhood years, the child explores, imagines, creates, imitates, experiences, reacts with others who offer the child the basic experiences that constitute faith at that time. In fun, wonder, hugs, caresses, they experience faith. A child putting the infant Jesus in the manger, taking part in a Christmas pageant, or joining in a friendship circle around a campfire in an outdoor setting are all participating in "experienced" faith. At that point, questions of belief and doctrine are not important.

Next comes "affiliative faith"—the faith of belonging, of being in community. The marks of this style are a rich sense of being a part, the dominance of religious affections, and a sense of authority. The faith community's story has authoritativeness and power. Corporate worship, a supportive cell group experience, being accepted into church membership as a youth—these and other experiences may contribute to a rich sense of "affiliative faith."

This is followed by "searching faith." Westerhoff has suggested, "In order to move from an understanding of faith that belongs to the community to an understanding of faith that is our own, we need to count and question that faith."[16] Some of the characteristics of this style are doubt, critical judgment, and the need to experiment and explore other lifestyles than one's own heritage. There is also awareness of the need to commit. Sometimes this leads to premature commitments to causes that will later seem unworthy of such loyalty.

The last ring in this tree of faith is "owned faith." When the needs of "searching faith" have been met, one moves into a new place. "Here, faith . . . becomes a central and vital part of the person's total being."[17] Such persons still have questions but are willing to stand on what they believe. They want to put their faith into personal and social action. They will be ready to communicate that faith in word and deed.

This process may be visualized in this overview of one's "tree of faithing."[18]

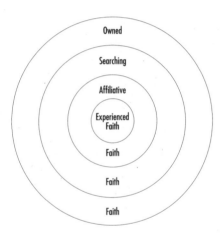

Westerhoff points out that though persons often see the movement from searching to owned faith as "conversion," really this whole process of faith development is conversion.[19]

JAMES FOWLER
Stages of Faith

James Fowler offers the most comprehensive and researched view of this process. After interviewing hundreds of persons, he has gained a perspective on the evolving structure of people's faith.

Fowler sees faith as a process of becoming. He believes that this process is:

growing in complexity,
sequential, the stages following after one another in a lifetime, and invariant, coming in the same order for all persons.

Fowler describes six possible stages of faith, though very few people pass through all six. Many stop much earlier than that. Here, then, are the six stages as Fowler views them.

Stage 1: Intuitive-Projective Faith (The Innocent). (The simpler, more dramatic terms in parentheses for each of Fowler's stages come from Charles McCullough.[20]) This may occur in preschool or early elementary years. This a time when life is fantasy-filled. The child constantly encounters new objects and experiences. The child imitates important adults, and is greatly affected by their examples, moods, actions, and stories. There is fluidity of thought and active imagination to make sense of one's world. Still, it is primarily a faith understood through the family experience.

Stage 2: Mythic-Literal Faith (The Literalist). This may begin at age six and continue to eleven or twelve, or it may continue through a lifetime. The child takes on the stories, beliefs, and observances that belong to her or his community. Beliefs, moral rules, and attitudes are interpreted literally. Symbols are also seen as one-dimensional and literal in meaning.

Stage 3: Synthetic-Conventional Faith (The Loyalist). This begins in adolescence and is also the stage where many adults find themselves. While a person brings together much more complex values and information, it is mostly a conformist stage. The person structures the ultimate environment in interpersonal terms. A person may not have a sure enough grasp of his or her own identity or independent judgment to feel free to construct a unique perspective. Belonging to a significant group is what is most important. And so the person is carefully attuned to the expectations and judgments of important others.

Stage 4: Individuating-Reflexive Faith (The Critic). This stage may come in one's teens, twenties, thirties, forties, or—for many people—never.

A person begins to reject the family faith, worship practices, beliefs. It involves doubting, struggling with new ideas and beliefs. It may take forms upsetting to others around the person, such as trying an extremely different belief system, a cult, or atheism. One may experiment politically at the same time. A person is taking responsibility for her or his own commitments, beliefs, attitudes, and lifestyle. This is not a comfortable stage. A person usually does not stay in it for lengthy periods, although there are a few who settle in at this stage. Such persons become the "loyal opposition," the iconoclasts, the "no" votes.

Stage 5: Conjunctive Faith (The Seer). This is a stage that is rarely approached before age thirty. It becomes a possibility in one's midlife or later years, but it is rather rare even there. One builds on and integrates the faith journey through stages 1–4, coming to an understanding of faith that is uniquely one's own. A person may be surprised to discover himself or herself reclaiming symbols, stories, and myths in his or her heritage that had been rejected. These treasures are reclaimed in a new way. Perhaps one has absorbed "the sacrament of defeat" and understands the reality of irrevocable commitments and acts. One comes to an understanding of paradox—the ability to unify opposites in mind and experience. A person may want to know more about the beliefs and practices of other faiths. Conviction, tolerance, and peace with what one claims as one's own out of one's faith heritage are all woven together in this stage of life.

Stage 6: Universalizing Faith (The Saint). This stage is experienced by only a few rare individuals. Fowler has noted that this is the stage that fascinates people the most, but about which he knows the least, for there are so few. These persons have a vision of an ultimate environment that includes all being. The person senses a call to be incarnator and actualizer of the ideal that envisions an inclusive and fulfilled human community. Fowler notes, "Many persons in this stage die at the hands of those whom they hope to change. Universalizers are often more honored and revered after death than during their lives. The rare persons who may be described by this stage have a special grace that makes them seem more lucid, more simple, and yet somehow more fully human than the rest of us. Their community is universal in extent."[21] Inclusiveness of all in their vision of community; radical commitment to justice and love; selfless passion for a transformed world—these are the marks of a stage 6 person.

SAM KEEN
The Passionate Life: Stages of Loving

Sam Keen has sketched out an alternative view of this process. He suggests that there are five stages on the way to the fullest kind of human life. These may be seen as stages of faithing or of loving.

First is *the child*, who is dependent and who wants to be with others. The child's primary word is "yes."

Next is *the rebel*, who is counterdependent, the opposite of the child. The rebel's primary word is "no."

Third, there is *the adult*, who can say both "yes" and "no." The adult knows the good and evil of culture, but has the dominant characteristic of cooperation. Keen notes that this is where most people end this journey. However, for the few who go beyond this to "the far side of character beyond culture's crust," there may be two more stages.

The outlaw begins with a crime, the killing of old authorities. This is part of a quest for autonomy beneath the roles and duties that have governed the adult. After half a lifetime, the fledgling outlaw wants to "explore the plurality, the madness, the uncontrolled forces that have previously been held in check by the character armor" of the adult.[22] In all this, the quest is to discover "What do I *really* want?"

In time, the person feels the limitations of the outlaw stage, for it is a lonely place. One needs communion and companionship to share life's ecstasies. *The lover or the fool* is the stage beyond outlaw. Vulnerability, compassion, childlikeness, mystery are a part of this time of life. Time becomes an open story. Hope grows strong. It is a life that is open to and filled with grace.[23]

These theories contain unique ideas, although they have a good bit in common as well. We can summarize them in a chart.[24]

Westerhoff	Fowler (McCullough)	Keen
Experienced Faith	Stage 1: Intuitive-Projective Faith (The Innocent)	The Child
Experienced Faith	Stage 2: Mythical-Literal Faith (The Literalist)	
Affiliative Faith	Stage 3: Synthetic-Conventional Faith (The Loyalist)	
Searching Faith	Stage 4: Individuative-Reflective Faith (The Critic)	The Rebel
Owned Faith	Stage 5: Conjunctive Faith (The Seer)	The Adult The Outlaw
Owned Faith	Stage 6: Universalizing Faith (The Saint)	The Lover or Fool

I Examine My Freedom to Search and to Doubt

Those who feel a tug toward a broader, more mature faith may have noticed something striking in these theories. Traditionally, religions and religious leaders have not encouraged doubts or searching. Faithful church members have often thought they were "losing their faith" if questions or doubts persisted with them for long. Though there is not quite a "Thou must *not* doubt or question" commandment, it sometimes feels like it.

By contrast, all three of the faith development theories I mentioned note the importance of doubt and searching for a fully developed faith. It is almost as if these theorists have a new commandment, "Thou *must* doubt and search, if thou wish to grow."

We live a in world of great mobility and in an age of information explosion. Knowledge is growing so fast in so many areas of life that most people need to commit to lifelong learning just to keep up. Can one's faith keep abreast of such changes and be an adequate guide in this kind of world? Or will it become some sort of quaint antique?

In this kind of world, many are not sure how to keep current in faith, or whether it is possible. Kenneth Stokes tells of Chuck, a man who was invited to join a church. He responded, "I'm not sure I'm ready to be a member of the church. . . . The older I get, the more confused everything is. Hell, I'm asking questions now I never even *thought of* in confirmation class."[25]

I believe that doubting and searching are a vital and important part of the religious journey. Those religious leaders who have been unresponsive to earnest doubters have ignored much of their own religious heritage. Certainly in Hebrew and Christian scriptures, we find Jeremiah doubting his calling, and Job crying out that he wished he knew where he could find God. There are psalmists who speak of their search, "My God, my God, why have you forsaken me?" (Ps. 22:1). Jesus prays that, if possible, the cup be passed from him. Thomas finds it hard to believe that Christ is alive, and then bows in wonder and worship.

Not only the Bible but history since those times reveals many great leaders who dared to doubt, question, challenge established beliefs and traditions. This list includes Augustine, Joan of Arc, Martin Luther, Abraham Heschel, Albert Schweitzer, Dietrich Bonhoeffer, Hans Küng, and many others.[26]

Nearly thirty years ago, Leslie Weatherhead confronted this issue in his provocative book, *The Christian Agnostic*. He pointed out that a Christian is one who is attracted to Christ. An agnostic is one who does not know, who has questions and is searching. Weatherhead suggested a "Christian agnostic" is "a person who is immensely attracted by Christ and who seeks to show his spirit, to meet the challenges, hardships, and sorrows of life in that spirit, but who, though he is sure of many Christian truths, feels he cannot honestly . . . 'sign on the dotted line'. . . to every aspect of some creed or doctrine."[27] Another great Christian leader of the last generation, Samuel Shoemaker used to urge people to be patient with their doubts and searchings. He simply invited persons to "commit as much of yourself as you are able to as much of God as you believe in."

In the inner journey of faith can one doubt, question, search? Yes, if that is what the journey demands. Indeed it may well be vital to the health of one's faith.

I Am Open to Serendipities That Aren't on the Road Maps

The road maps of faith development we have been discussing may not fit all of us. Some of us may be uncomfortable with the use of "stages" to describe such a process, and may be more comfortable with the image of a journey, a voyage, or something else. Hopefully these constructs have stirred thinking about where each of us is on our faith journey—and where would we like to be. At the same time, these road maps miss some oases, some places of beauty and growth on the journey. I want to be open to those delights of the spirit as well.

For example, as I reflect on my own journey of faith in the light of these theories, I note a number of places where they name experiences that were necessary and important for my personal growth. These theories help me understand how vital to my growth was a period of serious doubt and searching. The faith development people also remind us how comfortable each stage can be, and how unstable and frightening is the time when we are between stages. This in turn helps me understand resistance to change and to new insights—both in others and in me. As I will point out shortly, these faith development concepts give some understanding of why people choose different kinds of churches, and what are the varying tasks of church leaders in each of those churches.

On the other hand, the faith development theories deal with only part of my reality and miss some important aspects. For example, here are some of the other places where I have experienced discovery and growth:

- Occasionally, I have encountered another person and in some mysterious way, "deep spoke unto deep." I think of a time when I heard a person speak of a pioneering ministry. I was so drawn to him that for the first time I inwardly understood those Bible accounts where Jesus would look a person in the eye and say "follow me," and the person would do it! That was exactly how I felt. It was not that this person was so dynamic—as a matter of fact, he spoke slowly, reflectively, sometimes hesitatingly. I simply felt the connectedness, the integrity of who this person was and what he stood for. With variations, this has happened to me a few times since. I want to be open to the adventure and growth that I may experience when I encounter that mysterious appeal of a deeply spiritual person.

- I have experienced growth spurts when I took seriously the advice of the great missionary William Carey, "Attempt great things for God, expect great things from God." Sometimes this has meant giving more of my time, my abilities, my financial resources than I have before. Other times this means stretching for abilities I didn't know I had in order to fulfill what I felt called to do. Then, at times it means going into unknown territory because I feel so led. A few months after I write this, I will go do volunteer service with students in two Asian countries I have never visited before. I tremble in anticipation at what I may receive and what I may give on this adventure.

- Growth has awaited me when I have moved beyond the routine in my prayer and devotional life. I am stimulated to recognize that prayer is a natural impulse, an invitation to friendship with the divine. At the same time, there is something within me that resists this enriching, always available practice. I am helped by reading the devotional literature of persons—both contemporary and historical—who share discovery and invite deeper contemplation. A covenant with one or more persons that we will read the same book on spirituality in the same time frame sometimes gives me a needed discipline. With this mutual support and prodding, I made my way through ultimately rewarding devotional reading that I otherwise would have set aside.

- A deeper knowledge, a fresh encounter with the sacred scriptures is another source of spiritual refreshment. Centuries ago, a promise was made to persons leaving for the American colonies—that God has more light and truth yet to break forth out of God's holy word. I am amazed how often that promise is kept when I do disciplined individual or group study. In scripture I read the faith journeys, the searchings, the assurance of God's presence in suffering, the call to holistic mission. All this and more feeds my soul and grounds me for what I face.

- There are so many other opportunities of which I could speak. There is a connection between beauty and spiritual growth. Whether the beauty is in a sunset, a flower, a painting, or a piece of music, that beauty is an invitation to the spirit to soar. Some find their growth in journaling—in a faithful discipline of writing their joys and pains, searchings and discoveries for their eyes alone. Others find striking self-discovery in their dreams—recorded, reflected upon, and discussed.[28]

This suggests that while the faith development theories we mentioned give a broad framework and structure, there are other fascinating opportunities for spiritual growth and discovery that they don't include. I have mentioned a few of these, but my list is far from exhaustive.

I Consider Whether to Be "Spiritual" or "Religious"

Increasingly many folks are drawing a distinction between being "religious" and being "spiritual." When this differentiation is made, "religious" refers to being a part of worship practices, doctrines, structures, and programs of the church. People are seen as religious to the extent that they participate faithfully in the programs and organizations of a church.[29]

"Spiritual" implies the personalization or individualization of religion. One's quest is mostly a private one. Faith is nurtured through prayer, meditation, significant books, searching talks with a few persons one trusts, the beauty of art, music, and nature. Kathy, a person interviewed in a faith development survey, put it this way, "If I really want to communicate with my God, it's through people and through nature and not through church. . . . No, I don't find it there. Definitely through people."[30]

Among the younger of us midlife persons—the baby boomer

contingent—there has been a strong trend toward spirituality that avoids religiosity. In a 1988 survey conducted by *Rolling Stone* magazine, it was revealed that:

- 50 percent of respondents said they are less involved in organized religion than they expected to be, and
- 42 percent said that they are more interested in spirituality than they had expected they would be, while
- 72 percent felt that the diminished emphasis on religious training for children is a change for the worse.[31]

That survey seems to summarize a generation's ambivalent feelings about the "institutional church" (a dry, deadly description, if there ever was one). The response seems to be, "There are parts of 'religious' church life that do not speak to me; however, there are places (such as training for my children) where I do need help." For some, the dichotomy may be even stronger, "I feel betrayed by 'institutional religion' and yet I don't know where to turn for help in my search for spiritual values."[32]

In some ways, this "lover's quarrel" with the "institutional church" is nothing new. Persons of every age have often struggled with personal spiritual dilemmas and may have found the church more hindrance than help. Hundreds of years ago, a medieval writer suggested, "The church is like Noah's ark. If it weren't for the storm outside, I couldn't stand the smell inside." What was different in earlier generations was that, for the most part, persons carried on those struggles within the church. They tried to awaken the church to be more sensitive to persons such as they.

In the present, more are abandoning the church and carrying on a spiritual quest alone, or with occasional selected experiences.

I would hope that persons can choose both to be "religious" and "spiritual" and that they can hold these in healthy tension each with the other. That is where my journey takes me. I need a faith community, but one that has room for my searching and that encourages my spiritual quest. The person on a spiritual quest should hold his or her faith community accountable to be in touch and responsive to that search.

I Decide Whether I Need a Faith Community, and If So, Which One

I also hope people will see the value in joining together in communities. They can help each other nurture each other's children. Further, they can work together on tasks, missions, and issues that are too big for an individual or family to face alone. At the same time, they may need to challenge entrenched beliefs and rigid structure that has grown with the years. They may need to call the church to repentance for past betrayals.

If one agrees that a faith community and some organization is useful, then another question occurs: Of what faith community should I be a part?

Earlier in this chapter, we noted theories of the faith stages of individuals. There are also churches and religious groups that remain each of these faith stages. They see that particular stage as the way belief ought to be. Some of these may discourage one from moving beyond that stage, seeing it as a fall from grace. For example:

- There are churches in Fowler's stage 2, "The Literalist." Such churches interpret the Bible literally, teach persons what the Bible says and what to believe about it. For persons wanting a "black and white with no shades of gray" life view, this feels firm and reassuring. However, if that does not satisfy, a person may feel stifled.

- There are also churches in Fowler's stage 3, "The Loyalist." These churches advertise themselves as "The place to belong," or, "The end of your search for a friendly church." Most persons that Fowler interviewed were in stage 3, so this style of church life is widespread. (At least the attempt to be a warm, inclusive community is widespread. Some churches succeed at it more than others.) There may be an implied rule in such churches, "If you have a radical doubt or a searching question, please keep it to yourself. Don't upset the peace around here."

- There are a few churches that attempt to offer opportunities to explore Fowler's stages 4, 5, and 6, the critic, seer, and saint. I must admit these are too few and are found only in isolated places, even within the churches that aspire to provide this sort of environment. I don't mean to be overly critical of churches. Few people admit to wanting this kind of growth, so it is difficult to create opportunities. The church I serve offered a small group where there would be opportunity to raise all our searching questions and doubts. We advertised this opportunity widely, invited, recruited—and found eight persons in a congregation of five hundred! However, the eight of us had a stimulating series of discussions. The person wanting a church that will encourage this level of faith development might look for these signs: (1) in worship, an attitude of witness rather than dogmatism; (2) willingness of leaders and members to respond to questions, to admit failures, to share searchings; (3) prayer for, cooperation with, openness to other religious groups; (4) a network of small "cell" groups and/or "support" groups where one may meet some people who will spend enough time together that they may become honest with each other about their journeys; (5) a sense of mission, purpose, worthwhile things to do as an individual and community.

I Decide What I Mean by "Spiritual Growth"

Once we recognize our need for personal spirituality and community support, there is another question. What do we mean by spiritual growth? For most of us, "spiritual growth" relates to a pressing need, a problem, or a growing edge. It is that for which we need resources beyond ourselves in the present moment. When we experience progress or relief on the present issue, other opportunities loom before us. Spiritual growth is like walking toward the horizon. When we reach the one we see now, still another beckons to us, and another and another. This is true as long as we live. And so a vital question for each of us is, "Where am I in my spiritual journey, and what is my most pressing spiritual need right now?"

For some of us, this need might be finding help to do battle with an addiction. Something has mastered us. We are in its chains. This may be alcohol, other drugs, tobacco, food, sex, or something else. We may become aware that at times in our lives we become abusers—emotional, physical, sexual—of spouse or children. We may absorb abuse without resisting or escaping.

None of these chains is easily shed. Attempting to overcome these behaviors is an intense spiritual battle. It is good and necessary to have help at one's side in doing this. Counselors, caring friends and family, and twelve-step recovery groups may be means by which one claims outside strength.

If you suspect that you have one of these problems—or if trusted people tell you that you do—it is wise to seek help and begin work on it. Very likely, no other spiritual vista will beckon until that one is faced.

Others of us may have a different spiritual growth issue. Many of us—again a larger portion among the younger "baby boomer" group—may have left our churches at an early age or never took part. This was a dominant trend in our culture when we were growing up.

And so we may have what feels like embarrassingly elementary questions about religious faith. What does this religious group teach? What are its sacred writings? How does one handle them? Where does one start? And what does this mean to us now?

Those are all wonderful questions! People searching out the basics have a freshness, an excitement that enriches self and others. Persons of long faith heritage are privileged to respond to persons who ask these questions with interest and urgency. However, too often, a pair of mistakes are made. The spiritual novice finds it hard to admit this and to state her or his spiritual growth needs. That's one mistake. The other is that church leaders assume that this novice is more grounded. And so they put the person to work, teaching Sunday School or giving other leadership. The person may not be ready for this responsibility. Too often, this blocks further spiritual growth and contributes to the person feeling empty and burned out. Eventually such a person will probably drop out.

It is much wiser for the person and the community to be open with each other about spiritual pilgrimage. Growth and service can proceed in a way that is fulfilling rather than frustrating.

When we have mastered some basics—for example, overcoming addictions and knowing the basic teachings of our faith—there are other questions about what we mean by spiritual growth. There are those who challenge us to think of spiritual growth even more broadly than I have suggested. For example, M. Scott Peck, in *The Road Less Traveled*, writes, "I make no distinction between the mind and the spirit, and therefore no distinction between the process of achieving spiritual growth and achieving mental growth. They are one and the same."[33] Peck makes a powerful case for seeing the person as a whole. He contends that the spirit is not a separate part of the person, but a reality that pervades the whole. For Scott Peck, spiritual growth, mental growth, and mental health growth are one and the same.

Pastoral psychologist Howard Clinebell carries this a step further. He calls for holistic growth and suggest that there are six facets of such growth:

1. *Inner Growth: Enlivening One's Mind.* This includes intellectual growth, openness to oneself, self-esteem, creative interdependency, freshness of perception, richness of feelings (including both joy and pain), openness to newness and change, playfulness, creativity, and more.

2. *Inner Growth: Revitalizing One's Body.* This includes increasing awareness of mind-body wholeness, feeling more at home with our bodies, acceptance of our bodies beyond society's superficial valuing of the young and the beautiful, enjoyment of body pleasures, attention to the body's needs and care for the body's health.

3. *Renewing Our Relationships.* This includes strengthening and enriching our intimate relationships, committing ourselves to each other's growth, discovering and affirming our membership in each other, recognizing and learning to deal with relationships that are destructive, conflicted, or growth blocking.

4. *Growth in Relating to the Biosphere.* This means growing in our ecological awareness, caring for our biosphere, discovering all its inhabi-

tants as companions to be respected, cared for, enjoyed. It also involves learning to be renewed by nature and committing oneself to a partnership with nature. This means one will do one's part in overcoming our present ecological crisis.

5. *Growth in Relationships to Organizations and Institutions.* This involves enhancing our relationship with organizations, helping such to deal with the rigidity that stifles humanity, and dealing with them in ways to help them be more flexible and growth producing. This will lead one to such issues as economic injustice, racism, sexism, ageism, militarism, and nationalism.

6. *Spiritual Growth.* Clinebell notes that "Spiritual growth intersects the other five dimensions and is their unifying bond. Spiritual growth is at the heart of all human growth because it has to do with those things that clearly define us as being distinctively human. Spiritual growth aims at the enhancement of our realistic hope, our meanings, our values, our inner freedom, our faith systems, our peak experiences, and our relationship with God."[34]

If we accept Clinebell's view of spiritual growth, it is not only an area of life to be nurtured, it is also that vitalizing force that gives us strength to work on every issue we have mentioned in this book and more!

I like that view. More and more it has become the way I think about spiritual growth. It awakens me to areas where I have more growing to do. Each reader will have to decide what she or he means by spiritual growth and what beckons in the present moment.

I Resolve to Give of Myself

I have learned something from living this much of my life: I have something to give and the urge to give it. This is the stage of life where, as Erik Erikson told us in the first chapter, a basic life issue is "generativity versus stagnation." I can either cling to my achievements and ideas or I can listen to an inner voice to use my gifts in radical new ways on behalf of others.

I have discoveries to share, gifts to give, causes to support. There may be younger colleagues or friends who are interested in sharing my experience and wisdom.[35]

Perhaps I need to do some reengaging and conversations about my reconsidered and rediscovered faith and values with members of my own family unit first. At the same time, gift-giving of myself, my influence, my faith, my vision should not stop there. There may be others that will be interested as well.

One of my favorite sayings is this: "Every adult needs a child to teach. That's the way adults learn!" My inner growth will be more complete when I claim this growth enough to give some of it away—in generative mentoring.

In her book *Gift from the Sea*, Anne Morrow Lindbergh describes the middle years as a time of shedding shells—the shells of ambition, ego, and possessions, for example. Some of this shedding is scary and feels like death. However, she holds out the possibility that it can be the means of liberation by which we become more truly ourselves. She writes, "One is afraid. Naturally. Who is not afraid of pure space—that breath-taking empty space of an open door? But despite fear, one goes through the room beyond." She goes on to ask, cannot midlife be a time when we are finally free for enhancing the inner life, mind, heart, potential talent? Is this not the time to be free at last for spiritual growth?[36]

In this chapter I have named some of these opportunities for middle adults as to inward growth. As our exploration moves toward closure, there is one more topic to consider. What is one to believe? What beliefs still stand after the tests of living? What beliefs have been enhanced? What sustains? It is to that exploration that we will turn in the concluding chapter.

For Personal or Group Reflection and Discussion

1. At what times in your life have you tried to fulfill others' expectations of you (perhaps expectations that did not fit)? What has aided your clearer self-understanding?

2. Do you recognize dreams that you have had for your life?

What has happened to those dreams? How do you feel about this result?

3. As a midlife person, what seems more complex, vague, ambiguous to you now than it did fifteen or twenty years ago?

4. Does the author's contention about downward economic mobility, loneliness, rootlessness, depression ring true with you? What are your resources for coping?

5. Name the friends and groups that enrich your life. Do you need other friends? Other groups?

6. How would you describe your faith at the present moment? How does it differ from the faith you had as a youth?

7. How comfortable are you with raising hard questions or expressing doubt about your faith? Do you have questions/doubts you'd like to discuss and explore? If so, what are they?

8. Would you describe yourself as more "spiritual" or more "religious"? Why do you answer as you do?

9. What would you like to be your next step in spiritual growth?

10. In what ways do you plan to give of yourself as a midlife person? In what ways are you already doing so?

Resources

Brewi, Janice, and Anne Brennan. *Midlife: Psychological and Spiritual Perspectives.* New York: Crossroad, 1982.

Carroll, L. Patrick, S.J., and Katherine Marie Dyckman, S.N.J.M. *Chaos or Creation: Spirituality in Mid-life.* Mahwah, N.J.: Paulist Press, 1986.

Clinebell, Howard. *Growth Counseling.* Nashville: Abingdon, 1979.

——. *Well Being.* San Francisco: Harper, 1992.

Fisher, Kathleen. *Autumn Gospel: Women in the Second Half of Life.* New York: Paulist Press, 1995.

Fowler, James W. *Stages of Faith.* San Francisco: Harper and Row, 1981.

Fowler, James, and Sam Keen. *Life Maps: Conversations on the Journey of Faith.* Waco, Tex.: Word Books, 1978.

Keen, Sam. *The Passionate Life: Stages of Loving.* New York: Harper and Row, 1983.

McCullough, Charles. *Head of Heaven, Feet of Clay*. Cleveland: The Pilgrim Press, 1981.

Miller, Craig Kennet. *Baby Boomer Spirituality: Ten Essential Values of a Generation*. Nashville: Discipleship Resources, 1992.

Olson, Richard P. "Personal Becoming and Life Stages." *Baptist Leader* 46, no. 6 (Sept. 1984). Valley Forge, Pa.: Judson Press.

Parker, Dorothy. *The Portable Dorothy Parker*. New York: Viking Press, 1954.

Peck, M. Scott. *The Road Less Traveled*. New York: Simon and Schuster, 1978.

Roof, Wade Clark, et al. *A Generation of Seekers: The Spiritual Journeys of the Baby Boom Generation*. San Francisco: Harper, 1993.

Roschen, John Franklin. *Baby Boomers Face Midlife: Implications for Faith Communities in the '90's and Beyond*. Minneapolis: Adult Faith Resources, 1991.

Stokes, Kenneth. *Faith Is a Verb*. Mystic, Conn.: Twenty-Third Publications, 1989.

Weatherhead, Leslie. *The Christian Agnostic*. Nashville: Abingdon, 1965.

Westerhoff, John. *Will Our Children Have Faith?* New York: The Seabury Press, 1976.

Whitehead, Evelyn Eaton, and James D. Whitehead. *Seasons of Strength: New Visions of Christian Maturing*. New York: Doubleday and Company, 1984.

10

Credo of a Midlife Christian

"**R**EADY OR NOT, here I come!"—so we called out when we were "it" during a game of hide-and-seek we played in our childhood.

"Ready or not, here I come!"—something says to us sometime during the middle third of our life. Being middle aged is not an act of will. Rather, midlife is an experience that happens to each of us. It probably happens to each of us a number of times, sometimes with more force than others.

Janice Brewi writes, "One does not choose the mid-life experience any more than the twenty-month-old chooses to join the ranks of the 'terrible twos.' A new stage of physical or psychological growth arises in us, chooses us, as it were. The time is now."[1]

In midlife, we have work to do—faith work! David J. Maitland has aptly suggested that life stages are God's curriculum. There is "divine initiative to be discovered during the life process."[2] In the obstacles, conflicts, and problems one encounters in each life stage, there are valuable lessons to be learned. He continues, "It is for such reasons as these that progress through the life stages is not optional for Christians. No other experiences hold comparable potential for enhancing appreciation of one's humanity and for driving ever deeper the roots of one's humanity."[3] He contends, therefore, that the progressive work of the life stages is an "inescapable obligation/opportunity" for those who claim the Christian faith. Certainly we need faith resources to do the inner growing of which we spoke in the preceding chapter.

We need to find that faith perspective that gives a foundation for this particular period of our lives. We have questions to ask and resources to claim for the pressing life issues that are upon us. Some have found the faith of their childhood and youth wanting in such a time. Perhaps they turn to another major religion, to New Age possibilities, or something else.

I have been drawn to a rethought, reprayed, restruggled claiming of a historic Christian faith. As I reconsider this faith perspective, I discover that I had inserted some false promises and assurances that were not there, of which I needed to be relieved. I become aware of Christian teachings and themes that glow with new power and relate specifically to my midlife questions and needs. I see it again for the first time!

And so I offer you my "credo of a midlife Christian." It arises out of conversations with many midlife Christians and a study of scripture. Most of all it arises out of my own inward life of faith as I deal with the issues of this time in my life.

I put it before you as an invitation. May it help you to look inside to discover what you believe in your heart of hearts about the God of gods.

I Believe in a Personal God

Through much of my life, I have claimed the 139th Psalm as my favorite. This psalm becomes more important to me every year. It begins, "O God, you have searched me and known me. You know when I sit down and when I rise up; you discern my thoughts from far away. You search out my path and my lying down, and are acquainted with all my ways" (Ps. 139:1–3).

I am drawn to a faith in a personal God even though there have been long periods of time when I failed to see any evidence of this.

I say it humbly, feeling I know less of God than many who share this belief claim to know.

That I must be less bold in this claim does not trouble me. With any satisfying human relationship, I am fascinated to discover new aspects of that person's personality year after year. There is much in the majesty and greatness of God that I do not know. I hope that this awareness is an empty cup into which new experiences and discoveries can be poured.

Of all the metaphors of God in scripture, Jesus' embracing the picture of father-mother God is the one that grips me most powerfully. The tenderness I feel for my children, and now for my grandchildren, enriches my feeling and comprehension. This in turn draws me back to the depths of my relationship to parent God. I believe in a personal God.

I Believe in a Communicating God

I say this cautiously. I hear others make what seems to me to be extravagant claims about what God has said to them. Some of the things people claim God said are just plain silly; others are questionable, evil, or destructive. I believe in a communicating God, but I also think that people have the power to deceive themselves and others. I have this same self-deceiving power and temptation. Therefore I need a method of the heart and mind to explore into the mind of God as well as God's will and guidance for me.

This is an item that needs careful attention. Persons at the younger end of the middle third of life may have been gone from religious groups for a while. When they come back, they may look for different means of God's communication than the ones that satisfy me. Craig K. Miller, who has written of the baby boomer search for spirituality, comments:

> It is ironic that the churches who were the most supportive of the civil rights movement, who were on the cutting edge of the feminist movement, who battled for inclusive language, and who were the most active in supporting human rights are now the churches

that are hurting the most. Why is it that as boomers searched for God, they found the most powerful churches of the '50s and '60s to be meaningless?[4]

Miller's thoughtful answer is that in the search for God, boomers sought something other than their parents' "beliefs in a God who was very logical, rational, upright, and socially acceptable."[5] Worship of this God was formal and "relegated the laity into penitent observers of ritual and practice."[6] The theology that informed the clergy was difficult to communicate with laity and increased the distance between pew and pulpit. All this resulted in a church that failed to meet religious needs. (Miller is writing of the church of his childhood and youth.)

When faith broke out among baby boomers in the 1970s, it was likely to be of a quite different style. The Jesus Movement of the '70s was a come-as-you-are, accepting, Christ-as-personal-savior revival. The new evangelists were young, but proclaimed an old-time, Bible-toting, witness-giving type of faith. They told people to turn on to Jesus and enter the joy. They assured people Jesus was coming soon.

Many turned to charismatic groups, finding God's immediacy and love in handclapping services of praise, punctuated by hallelujahs and often marked by speaking in tongues.

Miller tells of a baby boomer, Tal Brooke, who felt that in his visits to many churches he had failed to find "the love that is so enthrallingly reported in the New Testament Church." After a long search for God, which took him to India for a time, he walked into Calvary Chapel in California. He recalled that he "felt an abundant flow of love the moment I walked through the door. There was not even a fleeting hint of judgmentalism here. Rather I sensed a terrific sense of belonging." Miller concludes:

> The Jesus movement personified what boomers had been looking for all along, a personal experience of godliness that said, "I am important," "I count," "Jesus loves me."[7]

While this is a strong segment, it is by no means all of the baby boomer population. Yet another segment was drawn into, or at least influenced by, that group of practices and beliefs known as "New Age" religion. For example recent surveys reveal that 42 percent of Americans believe they have been in contact with someone who has died; 63 percent of all adults report having experienced ESP (extrasensory perception); and 35 percent of Americans said that they had had a mystical experience "feeling very close to a powerful, spiritual force that seemed to lift you out of yourself."[8]

C. Peter Wagner sees a common theme here. He suggests that New Agers and charismatic Christians share a worldview that there is supernatural power from outside human existence that is available to operate through humans indirectly and directly. Each movement names a different power as the source. Each is convinced that they have tapped divine, supernatural power.[9]

I am grateful to Craig Miller and his analysis. It tells me how deep this hunger is. It points out to me what people have in common as they carry on this search for living communication with their God. It reminds me to be ever attentive to this need when I minister to folks in the middle third of life.

And yet, the solution that Miller describes does not satisfy everybody. I am among those it does not satisfy. Indeed, I experienced some of the options he describes (fundamentalism, revivalism, charismatic movement) in the churches of my childhood and youth. I left *that* in search of a more satisfying, thoughtful faith perspective.

As I have searched for an alternative way to be open to God's communication of presence and will, here is what I have found. I begin with what has been called "general revelation." I can know a fair amount about God's being and intention for me from God's creation and the document that reports on God's revealing acts among God's people—the Bible. In dialogue with many others, I read the Bible to find basic teachings, themes, events. In this, I attempt to keep central what is central there, and not get bogged down in what is peripheral. I am quite aware that my perceptions enter into this selection of what is central in the Bible. I do not confuse my interpretation of the Bible with the Bible itself. This needs to be open to further discussion and possible correction. Very briefly, such reflection leads me to the convictions that:

- God is creator of incredible beauty and of mysterious, sometimes destructive power.
- God identifies with the pain of all God's people and calls upon God's people to "do justice, love mercy, and walk humbly with our God."
- God expressed God's nature most clearly in the unconditional abundant love that was revealed in Jesus' life, death, and resurrection. There is nothing in all creation that can separate us from this love. We are called to love one another and the world as we have been first loved.
- God calls each believer to minister, and to that end empowers each with unique gifts and fruits of God's spirit.

I have bet my life on these beliefs, that they are true and can be trusted. If no further revelation were granted me, there would be enough here by which to live life.

Still, each of us hungers for that more personal guidance within this general revelation. I believe that such means are available. In a moving passage, John Powell suggests that we have at least six antennae in our human anatomy for communicating with God. He writes:

Can God put a new idea directly and immediately into my *mind?* Can [God] give me a new perspective in which to view my life with its successes and failures, agonies and ecstasies? Can God put new desires into my *heart,* new strength into my *will?* Can [God] touch and calm my turbulent *emotions?* Can [God] actually whisper words to the listening ears of my soul through the inner faculty of my *imagination?* Can God stimulate certain *memories* stored within the human brain when the memories are needed?[10]

Powell points to ways by which my disciplined heart and mind can receive fresh revelation. Therefore, I am called to a wide variety of practices that will sensitize my "antennae." Prayer, meditation, contemplation, silence, journal writing, reflection, listening, and more, offer the possibility of hearing our communicating God.

One thing more. Scripture points out that often God called to persons out of history. I listen both to the history of my times and my own personal history. This personal history includes my journey through life and my midlife questions and struggles. I need to pay attention to this, my history. Revelation of God's call, God's intent for me, may be there as well.

I believe in a communicating, revealing God.

I Believe in a Silent, Mysterious God

I speak of a personal, communicating God, but God is not always available the moment I want to be in touch. There are substantial periods of my life when I had the general beliefs of which I spoke, and nothing more.

Sometimes I have understood the reason why all too well. There was pride, arrogance, some unconfessed sin—perhaps some unrecognized sin. These factors corroded my receiving antennae and left me alone. At other times, I have not understood the reason for this sense of absence and silence.

Eugene C. Bianchi has noted how the Christian contemplative tradition may be of help to the searching midlife person. In some ways this tradition parallels the midlife experience. He notes that in meditation one experiences a gradual movement away from active reasoning toward prayer. This in turn leads to a state of simplicity within one's soul. "This more passive, listening attitude of contemplation allows us to break through ego facades, experience genuine feelings within, and begin to unify self and world."[11] This in turn may lead to what has been called "infused contemplation" or "the prayer of silence." This may be described as an experience of emptiness or void. This is not an alarming void, but a "quiet emptiness" that may be filled "with calming peace and richness, which allows the broken strands of our existence to be mended and old wounds to be healed." These are not intentional, self-healing acts of reason, but gifts from beyond.

In the life of contemplation—paralleled by the midlife experience—there is another silence that is not so reassuring. Traditionally mystics speak of this as the "dark night of the soul."

> This experience of suffering is marked by aridity of spirit, confusion, and desolation. Meditation seems useless and tedious; the soul feels devoid of God's presence and consolation. The contemplative is tempted to abandon the whole enterprise. Nevertheless, with perseverance, a new level of peace, now chastened and more subtle, enters the soul.[12]

Bianchi reminds me that the terrifying absence/silence of God is a common experience. Those who seek God most ardently and live disciplined lives seeking to know that presence have such experiences. Misery loves company, and so this is a helpful reminder. Devout persons of the ages and the present experience God's absence as I sometimes do. They have discovered that though painful, it is a helpful part of one's life with God.

Faith development theorists suggest that doubt is a necessary step on the way to owned faith. The contemplative tradition tells us that experiencing God's absence may be necessary to know the joy of God's presence.

I believe in a God that is sometimes silent and always mysterious.

I Believe in a Community-creating God

So far I have been speaking of the individual's search for and experience of an intensely personal God. This must be balanced by another truth. The Bible describes God as community-creating, as one who loves and ardently seeks a group of people. In reading scripture, one will discern that God's passion for a community of people is at least as great as God's passion for individual believers.

God calls Abraham to found a nation that will be as numerous as stars in the sky or sand on the beach. Abraham is promised that through this nation all the nations on earth will be blessed. The generations pass. This people find themselves enslaved in Egypt.

God hears the cry of their suffering and sends the deliverer Moses, who leads them into the wilderness. God makes covenant with them and calls upon them to be God's people.

God's spokespersons, the prophets, constantly call the people of Israel back to this covenant relationship. Prophets call the people of Israel a faithless spouse, or a child that God taught how to walk without the child's even acknowledging it.

Over and over it is made clear that God eagerly desires a people who will be faithful, who will praise, worship, love, and serve God.

The New Testament states this theme in ever new ways. Jesus called many followers; he selected an inner circle of twelve not only to send them forth, but "to be with him" (Mark 3:14). They followed him, served and stayed with him. They were together when the resurrected Christ appeared to them, and again (with a larger group of followers) when God's spirit came upon them at Pentecost.

Over and again writers of the New Testament affirm God's high and holy intent for the people called together to follow Christ. These groups (local ones and as a universal totality) are called the body of Christ, the temple of God, the bride of Christ, the family of God, and much more. It is made clear that just as Jesus was a healing presence, so the church (whether gathered or scattered) is called to "be Christ" in the world.

William Barclay has contended that the New Testament knows nothing about a solitary Christianity, and that is certainly true. Scripture points to a community-creating, community-seeking God.

As I relate that scriptural teaching to my life, I see its significance. God has entrusted tremendous power to human relationships. Friendship, marriage, family, education, and other learning are all relationship experiences whose combined power have contributed much to what each person is, knows, and believes.

And so God has called into being the community of faith. Scripture reveals that God has done this for a variety of reasons:

- so that people may encourage one another through worship, praise, and personal care
- to mediate Christ's forgiveness and love each to the other
- to make the community that supportive place where, "If one member suffers, all suffer together with it; if one member is honored, all rejoice together with it." (1 Cor. 12:26)
- to witness both by its inward harmony and by its outward acts and words to the winsome invitation of Christ to all
- to go into the world and make disciples of all nations
- to do justice, love mercy, and walk humbly with our God

However, there's a problem. As we have noted, many people have looked for that kind of church and have not found it. People have come to church with those kinds of hungers and have not been satisfied.

Worse yet, people have been hurt by churches. Some have been deceived out of large amounts of money. Others have experienced the church as irrelevant to the troubling issues of the time—racism, sexism, and poverty. Many others have absorbed personal pains from other members or the church structure. This has led to disillusionment with the church. As I write, I have slowly healing scars over some fresh wounds received within a church.

This is a dilemma—a God who seeks community and a community of faith that falls far short of God's intent! What are we to make of this? While we cannot entirely resolve this scandal, there are some things that can be said: (1) the churches in New Testament times fell far short also. As a matter of fact, it was some of their greatest messes that led to some of Paul's most urgent calls to be the church Christ intends! (2) part of our disappointment comes because we have hoped for so much from the church; (3) at least some of the failure of the church is because of me: my late friend Dave, a deacon in a church I once served, used to tell each new member, "I have to warn you that you are joining an imperfect church—you see I am part of it"; (4) just as individuals have times of God's absence—"dark nights of the soul"—so do churches, and just as we keep persisting in our individual spiritual drought, we are called to be faithful through some puzzling and discouraging times in our community life; (5) I need to recall those relationships that have touched me most richly and recognize "that was part of the beloved community that God intends"; (6) God allows each rich variety as to what form of faith community one selects. One may find a little house church of ten, or a superchurch or denomination of hundreds of thousands. God loves and abides in each.

There is more I need to reason, discover, and do about the faith community. I can neither accept it as it is nor abandon it—I must maintain my lover's-quarrel tension with it. This is because I walk in relationship with a community-creating, community-seeking God.

I Believe in a Cosmic God

Those of us whose middle years occur in the 1990s or in the twenty-first century will experience "globalization" to a far greater extent than any previous generation on our planet.

A generation ago Marshall McLuhan spoke of our planet as a "global village," and it is becoming more so all the time. Cameras record and the media broadcasts the joys and agonies of the human family in every part of the earth. We witness and experience a confrontation in Tiananmen Square, the fall of the Berlin Wall, the collapse of communism, starving children and civil wars in numerous places. Some suggest that communism collapsed in Eastern Europe because the rulers could no longer control knowledge or information.

Globalization is also seen in the mobility and birth rates of the various groups of people. In the United States, from 1980 to 1990, the Asian population increased by 107 percent and the Hispanic population by 53 percent. Demographers predict that by the year 2010, 80 percent of children in Hawaii will be nonwhite. Many states will have a majority of nonwhite children, including New Mexico (77 percent), California (57 percent), Texas (57 percent), New York (53 percent), Florida (53 percent), and Louisiana (50 percent). In the District of Columbia 93 percent of children will be "minorities." In our most populous states, there is a pressing need for persons of many races, ethnic groups, and national origins to discover how to live together in harmony and peace.

There are global changes in population as well. In 1990, Asia contained half of the world's population. By the year 2000, it will have two thirds. Europe's percentage of the world population will have diminished to 6 percent.

These changes are seen in the worldwide Christian church as well. When Columbus came to the New World in 1492, 93 percent of the world's Christians were European. Theology, music, worship, and the arts merged Christian thinking with European culture. Today that is drastically changed and changing. In 1980, 31 percent of the world's Christians were European; this will shrink to 21 percent by the year 2000. North American Christians made up 14 percent of the world total in 1980; in 2000 it will be 10 percent. By contrast the percentage for Africa will increase from 12 percent to 17 percent; for East Asia it will increase from 1 percent to 7 percent.

It is estimated that in this twenty-year period the number of African Christians will grow from 164 million to 324 million. In East Asia the numbers will likely explode from 16 million to 128 million in 2000. The center of the vitality, power, and creativity of the Christian faith is shifting to Asia and Africa.[13]

There is another revolution going on at the same time—the feminization of society, including many of its institutions, and certainly including the Christian church. Far too slowly the unique leadership, perspective, and gifts of women are being recognized. Ordination of women has come to some denominations that formerly did not allow it. In some groups women have been chosen for bishoprics and other positions of church authority. Every branch of the theological discipline has been enhanced by formidable women scholars who have come to old subjects and issues with new eyes.

Yet another consciousness has dawned upon our generation. Perhaps it came most clear with that picture of an "earthrise" taken by the astronauts from the moon. That fragile, beautiful planet floating in space has come to be understood as "spaceship earth." Awareness rose that this "spaceship" needed attention and care.

Unfortunately, this awareness has not been matched by as great an effort as is needed. Spaceship earth is showing signs of strain. There are polluted water and air, toxic waste dumps, nuclear accidents, deforestation, erosion of the land, oil spills, holes in the protective ozone layer. Clearly, there is a need for a committed corps of people who love spaceship earth and who will make every effort to raise consciousness and allocate priorities for its care.

There is also a need for a theology that integrates the events and problems of which we are speaking. This theology needs to be a source of perspective and clear ethical thinking on these matters. In regard to the ecological crisis some have turned to Eastern or Native American religions, seeing them as more compatible with the care needed. Such persons see the biblical heritage, particularly God's statement to humans to "have dominion" over other species, as part of the problem.

I believe that this is a misinterpretation of the biblical teaching about creation and the care of the earth. Instead, I read those poetic accounts of creation where God sees that all that God has made is very good! (Gen. 1). I hear the psalmist, touched with the beauty of creation, exclaiming, "O God, our Sovereign, how majestic is your name in all the earth" (Ps. 8:1). I experience the prophet's dreams of a nature even more harmonious and productive. I hear a call to care for the earth because it is God's, because it is holy, and because we are but its temporary stewards.

Scriptures offer a perspective for globalization and feminization as well. Jesus lived in Palestine. An early convert was African. Christianity took root in Europe only because early Christian missionaries came *there*. However, much more basic than the ethnic roots of Christianity is the cosmic vision of why it even happened. Scripture affirms "God so loved the *world*" that God gave us Christ (John 3:16). "In Christ God was reconciling the *world* . . ." to God's self (2 Cor. 5:19). And so Paul could say, "There is no longer Jew or

Greek, there is no longer slave or free, there is no longer male and female; for all of you are one in Christ Jesus" (Gal. 3:28).

The contemporary Christian is called to continue the work of reconciliation that the early church began. The vast opportunities of today give us a chance to live out our God's dream and will. This dream is for harmony among humankind and between humankind and nature.

It has been noted that one of the gifts of midlife is that, at least once in a while, we can see 360 degrees—in all directions. We can absorb the images of a cosmic God and perhaps even interpret them to those before us and those after us. To be granted that vision, even temporarily, may be one of the spiritual gifts of midlife.[14]

I believe in a cosmic God.

I Believe in a Laughing God

There is a modest—but often ignored—theme in the Bible. This theme is always important, but perhaps especially so in our middle years. I point to the references that speak of a God of joy and laughter.

For example, when God speaks to Job out of the whirlwind, one of the questions God asks is, "Where were you when I laid the foundations of the earth? . . . when the morning stars sang together and all the heavenly beings shouted for joy?" (Job 38:4, 7). When God gives a child to Abraham and Sarah in their old age, Sarah exclaims, "God has brought laughter for me; everyone who hears will laugh with me" (Gen. 21:6). In turn she names her son "laughter" (a fair translation of "Isaac").

God's laughter is noted at least three times in the Psalms (Ps. 2:4, 37:13, and 59:8). Granted, the psalmists represent God as laughing in derision at the wicked. Still, the image of a God who laughs at all is a stretch!

Another psalm remembers a time when God's blessings were experienced, "Then our mouth was filled with laughter and our tongue with shouts of joy" (Ps. 126:2).

The writer of Proverbs makes clear that laughter is good for people. "A cheerful heart is a good medicine, but a downcast spirit dries up the bones" (Prov. 17:22).

When we look at Jesus, we need be aware that excellent Bible scholars see more humor and play in his life and teachings than we might have imagined. His playful exaggerations and his use of irony gave a light touch to the important truths he shared. Brewi and Brennan write, "I see in the Gospels a Jesus so playfully familiar with nature and the earthly dimension of life that he continually uses them in his teaching."[15] He said to his disciples, "I have said these things to you so that my joy may be in you, and that your joy may be full" (John 15:11). "I came that they may have life, and have it abundantly" (John 10:10b). Reflecting on this perspective of the gospel accounts, Brewi and Brennan write:

> I know a Jesus in the Gospels who played beautifully and respectfully with the law because he knew that it existed for him and for each of us, not we for it. . . . To be committed to this Jesus, each of us is called to be committed to his playful attitude toward life and death itself. . . . Jesus lived a spirituality of play. In everything he had an attitude of play and he freely played. His life from birth till death gives witness to an attitude of playfulness and a rhythm of playing and praying.[16]

This basic theme of a God of laughter and joy provides a needed perspective for us midlife persons, for me at least. Without such a perspective, I might become quite self-absorbed and self-important. Or, on the other hand, I am in danger of falling into despair over the great problems and heavy burdens midlife people face.

Belief in a laughing God leads the believer into at least two areas. One of these areas is story. Someone once said that God created humans because God loves stories! If I recognize my own story as one of those in which God delights, then I begin to see things there I might have previously missed. I see human quirks and foibles to be enjoyed with healthy doses of self-hilarity and ridicule. I see love and sustenance where at the time I saw only my struggle to survive. I see a person becoming and growing, touched by the love of God through the love of many persons. I'm glad that God loves stories, including my story.

Yet another area is that of play and humor. Pioneering psychologist Abraham Maslow believed that the ability to play was one of the ideal traits of the self-actualized personality—the fully functioning, fully alive person. He described playfulness as fun, joy, amusement, gaiety, humor, exuberance, and effortlessness. It is an attitude as well as an activity, a basic element of wholeness.

Norman Cousins claimed for us all the truth that laughter can both be part of the cure for illness (it was in his situation) and a sign of wellness: "A rhythm of laughter and fun running through our days will temper our single-minded seriousness and put us on the way to better well-being."[17]

Brewi and Brennan add that a basic element of living creatively is to play. In play, one can listen to one's inner self and imagine other ways of being. Humor gives the perspective that one can mock the serious business of the world and the mighty who carry it out. Humor and play are expressions of inner freedom. They conclude:

> If we are to be truly committed to our own growth in the second half of life we must be intent on making prayer and play a greater and greater reality in our life. . . . Praying and playing open for us possibilities for growth that we would never have dreamed of. Praying and playing allow us to trust and believe in the outcome for our existence even while we are on the way. Prayer and play allow us to imagine other ways of being, other orders and patterns of self and society. Prayer and play allow us to distance ourselves from the centrality of our causes, our work, our ministry, our preoccupations. Prayer and play open us to the other side of everything and to cure us of our terrible one sidedness. Prayer and play allow us to image other sides of self. . . . Prayer and play let us experience the Creator in new and unfathomable ways. Prayer and play connect us to the deep inner recesses of our personality. Prayer and play unite us to the world of people outside ourself, to

the glories of nature, and to the accomplishments of other generations and our own contemporaries. Prayer and play make my living and working more Godlike.[18]

The joys and mysteries of story, humor, and play are open to me. This is made possible by my belief in a laughing God.

I Believe in a God of Transformation, Resurrection, and New Birth

In the previous chapter we spoke of several dimensions of one's inner personal exploration: the search for a clearer self-understanding; an examination of one's dreams and hopes; and the naming of one's spiritual hungers, among others.

In that chapter we looked at the person's experience in exploring these topics. There is a theological dimension to this as well—the God of transformation is at work within us, bringing about renewal and change.

Bob Buford speaks of this needed transformation in modern sports terms. He describes midlife as "halftime." It is time to review the first half and plan strategy for the second half—of life. He notes that the first half has to do with getting and gaining, learning, and earning. That needed to be. But those who fail to stop for inner divine guidance about the second half, who simply try to repeat the first half, will be disappointed indeed. This was true of his experience. Though he was a fabulously successful businessman, he was haunted by questions of meaning, mission, purpose in life. At "halftime" he faced these questions, lived through the death of his only son, and asked friends and consultants to help him get in touch with life's most central purpose for him.

This led to a radical restructuring of his life. This included using his leadership skills to help churches be more effective. However, he sees this summons at halftime as more than an individual experience—it is a call of God to transformed living, a call that comes to all and which people avoid at their peril. If the call is heeded, the second half of life will involve living beyond the immediate. It will be about releasing divine creativity and wisdom through the yielded person.

Buford writes:

> Eventually, your first half will end. The clock will run out. If it happens unexpectedly—if you do not take responsibility for going into half time and ordering your life so that your second half is better than the first, you will join the ranks of those who are coasting their way to retirement. Your second half will be a slower version of the first, with fewer and fewer successes and very little significance. But if you take responsibility for the way you play out the rest of the game, you will begin to experience the abundant life that [God] intended for you.[19]

There is a Bible image that is often used to describe this transformation—rebirth. In the third chapter of John, Jesus tells a seeking leader named Nicodemus, "Unless one is born anew [one] cannot see the [dominion] of God." The incredulous Nicodemus asks, "How can [anyone] be born when [one] is old? Can [one] enter a second time into [the] mother's womb and be born?" Jesus responds, "Unless one is born of water and Spirit, [one] cannot enter the [dominion] of God" (John 3 RSV).

When Jesus says one must be born *again*, the word "again" translates the Greek *anothen*. Bible scholars note that in Greek, this word may have three different meanings: (1) from the beginning, and, therefore, completely, radically to one's foundations; (2) for a second time; (3) from above, and therefore from God.

Bible scholar William Barclay believes that all three meanings are included in Jesus' phrase "you must be born again," and that the term is therefore untranslatable in a single phrase. Instead, he suggests a translation that requires a complex sentence:

> To be born again is to undergo such a radical change that it is like a new birth; it is to have something happen to the soul which can only be described as being born all over again; and the whole process is not human achievement, because it comes from the grace and the power of God.[20]

Sometimes Christians speak of being "born again"—of having a vivid experience of spiritual rebirth through faith in the living Christ. That is a fitting use of the term. However, the symbol of rebirth images other midlife transformations as well.

For example, Iris Sangiuliano quotes the late poet Anne Sexton, "Women are *born twice*." Some are—Annie Sexton was one who was. She had never attended college, but had simply been someone's wife. Then, one day, she happened to hear some poetry. She thought, "I think I can do that!" and she did. Sangiuliano's study traces the path that women have taken toward a *second birth*. By this she means the emergence of an identity, a dream, a task that truly expresses who that woman is. It is the dawning of a woman's distinct identity, in and of herself, rather than an attached or ascribed identity—someone's wife or mother.[21] While this particular rebirth was probably more rare and more necessary when she wrote (the 1970s), the image holds true.

Indeed, Gail Sheehy happens on this same term rather unexpectedly in her most recent work on life stages. She tells that she conducted many "life history interviews" with famous and little-known people in preparation for this work, and asked herself what she learned:

> As I read over the transcripts of the hundreds of life history interviews I had done with women and men in middle life, a new theme, one of *surprise and rebirths*, was recapitulated loud and clear. More and more people were beginning to see there was the possibility of a *new life* to live, one in which we could concentrate on becoming better, stronger, deeper, wiser, funnier, freer, sexier, and more attentive to living the privileged moments, even as were also getting older, lumpier, bumpier, slower, and closer to the end.[22]

Brewi and Brennan, Christian Jungian psychologists, come to this imagery with a more specific theological point of view. They speak of midlife as:

> The third major birth that one encounters in the life cycle. It is a dying and a rising. Mid-life is a transpersonal moment in the per-

son's life as essential as the first and last transpersonal moments in the life cycle, being born and dying. The mid-life experience is the result of the human psyche entering a new phase of its development.[23]

These persons are saying that there is a life force—a divine force, if you will—toward a vigorous personal renewal in midlife. This force allows us to decrease our efforts at being a child or youth and move into an adult agenda. We no longer have to pretend that we are younger than we are. We may be freed from needing to conform to others' expectations. Each of us may therefore be free to discern what we want and, even more deeply, what God wants with the rest of our lives. People may learn to emphasize things they once avoided and to avoid things that once they emphasized. Evelyn Eaton Whitehead and James D. Whitehead put it vividly, "Adult maturity invites me to find a greater comfort with my own plural and unfinished self."[24]

While this transforming process can be inhibited, obstructed, or distorted, it is a force in one's life with which one must reckon. There is adventure in the air. The next chapter of life will be different. One is wise to be powerful and equipped for the journey. Persons of faith believe that both the call to change and the power to do so come from God.

I believe in a God of transformation, resurrection, and new birth.

I Believe in a God of Freedom and of Managership and of Mission

I have been describing a God who moves in history and in individual lives. This God reveals self and provides guidance and strength for wise living. This God was present at my birth and has led me forward through each stage of my life to the present. I believe that this God summons me to negotiate the needed midlife changes. As I attempt to do so, God will walk before me into this and the next stages of my life.

However, I see this through eyes of belief, having taken a leap of faith into this perspective. I do so freely, following my heart and head. I am not coerced by the God in whom I trust. I am granted the freedom to believe or not, to be open to God's revelation or not, to follow the leading I experience or not.

The Bible portrays a caring God who invites, knocks on our door and summons us—but who gives us the freedom to respond as we will. This is not to say that it is a matter of indifference how we respond. It is only to say that God grants us the freedom to respond as we will.

As a matter of fact, the Bible also portrays this God of freedom as a God of managership. I am responsible for managing all that is entrusted to my care.

One area for which I am to be a responsible manager is this experience of midlife itself! Eugene Bianchi has solemnly noted that "unless the inner conversions of middle age take place, there is little hope that elderhood will advance beyond the growing despair and selfish concerns attached to gradual decline."[25] We have seen cases where those conversions fail to happen. The most pathetic of midlife or older persons are those who refuse to admit and face the process of aging. Some terror of aging or death is probably the source of most behavior labeled as "midlife crazies."

I am called to a managership of my time, including the experience of growing, maturing, aging. Free under God to choose how to manage it, there are important consequences that result from my decision.

In midlife, each of us is manager of many things:

- a frail, mortal body, which by proper health practices can be effective and vigorous for a longer period of time
- 500 to 700 skills (remember?), including some vital ones that may be needed in today's world but which have not yet been discerned and developed
- relationships with a number of people
- revelations that may have been granted me and my faith response to God's communication with me

- calls of God from out of the history of our times, calls about the needs of God's world and God's suffering people
- employed and volunteer positions of leadership and influence
- the rest of my life

This aspect of theology responds to a longing felt by many people. Craig Miller sees this as a particular urgent hunger among baby boomers. He writes,

> As baby boomers search for God, what they desire more than anything else is to be part of a spiritual adventure that will challenge them, that will cause them to grow, that will throw off the old and bring in the new, that will engage them with the holiness and sanctity of life, that will put them in places where they will encounter the creative forces of the universe, that will lift them up from the grinding boredom to life to let them know they are unique and important, that their life has meaning and purpose. People desire to have a mission, an important goal toward which they are working.[26]

God reveals. God calls. God invites persons to be involved in the world's suffering and pain and thus to find meaning and significance in life. God gives us freedom to respond, but we are accountable for those decisions.

I believe in a God of freedom and of managership and mission.

I Believe in a God of Hope

There is so much change in our personal lives and in our world that we may tremble in confusion. There are such shifts in knowledge and in what society admires or disdains that we may be filled with anxiety. Even the church (especially the church!) is in ferment. Those of us who have tried to stay with it find changing concepts of worship, faithfulness, and meaningful contemporary programs.

I am attempting to formulate a credo to help me to walk through this stage of my life in this world. At the same time, I am trying to stimulate your thinking and believing. In doing so, I have had enormous amounts of change and issues on which to reflect.

However, there are parts of what I believe that do not change. One of those firm foundations is my belief in a God of hope. Biblical hope is that God is not ultimately defeated—confused and troubling as the present may appear. God's cosmic purposes are in God's hands and will ultimately be accomplished.

As it touches the individual believer, there are two dimensions of hope. One aspect is that "I shall see the goodness of God in the land of the living" (Ps. 27:13). This includes a confidence that while pain and sorrow are a part of living, that there are rich discoveries and an experience of God's sustaining presence in the midst of them. It also implies that when one is in a "down" time in life—personally, professionally, relationally, that there are better days coming. It is a confidence that help from beyond us will operate within us. As a Bible verse promises, "suffering produces endurance, and endurance produces character, and character produces hope, and hope does not disappoint us, because God's love has been poured into our hearts through the Holy Spirit that has been given to us" (Rom. 5:3b–5).

Christian hope also addresses one's finitude, one's eventual death. We are called to acknowledge that we do indeed age and will one day die. Then we are promised that the God who walks with us in life will walk with us in death.

Ashleigh Brilliant has a cartoon in which he says, "I hope it's a nice day—on the day after the day I die." In that statement is a gentle call to hope. After I die, God is still alive and active in God's world. Life goes on. I have moved on to a new stage of growth—my relationship with God in the glory that is yet to be revealed.

Christian hope recognizes that I am finite, and that is OK. It is God in God's providence and grace who has created life as it is. God has set the limits of human life. I will not accomplish all to which I aspire, but that is okay. I attempt to be responsible. I trust in the God revealed in the death and resurrection of Christ.

With eyes of faith and hope I believe that "neither death nor life . . . nor anything else in all creation will be able to separate us from the love of God in Christ Jesus our Sovereign" (Rom. 8:38–39).

"Therefore, my beloved, be steadfast, immovable, always excelling in the work of [God], because you know that in [God] your labor is not in vain" (1 Cor. 15:58).

I have shared my credo and filled it in with some of my provisional theology for being a midlife Christian in times such as ours. May this stimulate you to a rediscovery and a reclaiming of your foundational beliefs. For I will need your strength as you need mine. We are in this journey together.

For Personal or Group Reflection and Discussion

1. Write your personal midlife credo. Do so by finishing this sentence in as many ways as you wish: "I believe in a God of . . ." Compare this with the author's statements and with one another's. Look for points of contact and for unique perspectives.

2. In the middle third of your life, is your experience more of the communicating God or the silent God? Have you experienced both sides of this?

3. What have been the most spiritually enriching communities you have ever experienced? (These can be any size—one other person, small group, larger church or organization.) From that experience, what did you learn of the community-building God?

4. Do you share the author's belief in a "cosmic" God as he describes it? If so, to what concerns or causes is this God calling you?

5. Have you experienced a dancing, laughing God? Tell another about such experiences. Do you experience this aspect of God and of yourself as much as you want to? If not, what can you do to find yet more opportunities?

6. At what point does your obedience to God fill your need for mission, purpose, and adventure in life?

7. As you reflect on your faith, what gives you hope?

Resources

Barclay, William. *The Gospel of John*. Edinburgh: Saint Andrew Press, 1956.

Bianchi, Eugene C. *Aging as a Spiritual Journey*. New York: Crossroad, 1989.

Brennan, Anne, and Janice Brewi. *Mid-Life Directions: Praying and Playing—Sources of New Dynamism*. New York: Paulist Press, 1985.

Brewi, Janice, and Anne Brennan. *Celebrate Mid-Life: Jungian Archetypes and Mid-Life Spirituality*. New York: Crossroad, 1990.

————. *Mid-Life: Psychological and Spiritual Perspectives*. New York: Crossroad, 1982.

Buford, Robert P. *Halftime: Changing Your Game Plan from Success to Significance*. Grand Rapids, Mich.: Zondervan, 1994.

Fischer, Kathleen. *Autumn Gospel: Women in the Second Half of Life*. Mahwah, N.J.: Paulist Press, 1995.

Groeschel, Benedict J. *Spiritual Passages: The Psychology of Spiritual Development*. New York: Crossroad, 1992.

Maitland, David J. *Looking Both Ways: A Theology for Mid-Life*. Atlanta: John Knox Press, 1985.

Miller, Craig Kennet. *Baby Boomer Spirituality: Ten Essential Values of a Generation*. Nashville: Discipleship Resources, 1992.

Olson, Richard P. *Mid-Life: A Time to Discover, A Time to Decide*. Valley Forge, Pa.: Judson Press, 1980, 1982.

————. "Personal Becoming and Life Stages." *Baptist Leader* 46, no. 6 (Sept. 1984): 4–7.

Powell, John. *He Touched Me: My Pilgrimage of Prayer*. Niles, Ill: Argus Communications, 1974.

Roof, Wade Clark, et al. *A Generation of Seekers*. San Francisco: Harper, 1993.

Roschen, John Franklin. *Baby Boomers Face Midlife: Implications for Faith Communities in the '90's and Beyond*. Minneapolis: Adult Faith Resources, 1991.

Sangiuliano, Iris. *In Her Time*. New York: William Morrow, 1978.

Sell, Charles M. *Transitions through Adult Life*. Grand Rapids, Mich.: Zondervan, 1985, 1991.

Sheehy, Gail. *New Passages: Mapping Your Life Across Time*. New York: Random House, 1995.

Stokes, Kenneth. *Faith Is a Verb*. Mystic, Conn.: Twenty-Third Publications, 1989.

Whitehead, Evelyn Eaton, and James D. Whitehead. *Christian Life Patterns*. Garden City, N.Y.: Doubleday, 1979.

———. *Seasons of Strength: New Visions of Christian Maturing*. New York: Doubleday, 1984.

Notes

1. Other Maps of the Midlife Experience

1. Evelyn Eaton Whitehead and James D. Whitehead, *Christian Life Patterns* (Garden City, N.Y.: Doubleday, 1979), 29–30.
2. Iris M. Ford, *Life Spirals: The Faith Journey* (Burlington, Ont.: Welch Publishing, 1988, 1990), 90–91.
3. Erik Erikson, *Childhood and Society* (New York: W. W. Norton, 1950), 247–73.
4. Gwen Hawley, *Measures of Psychosocial Development* (Odessa, Tex.: Psychological Assessment Resources, 1988).
5. Matthew Linn, Dennis Linn, and Sheila Fabricant, *Healing the Eight Stages of Life* (New York: Paulist Press, 1988).
6. Daniel Levinson, Charlotte N. Darrow, Edward B. Klein, Maria H. Levinson, and Braxton McKee, *The Seasons of a Man's Life* (New York: Alfred A. Knopf, 1978), 19.
7. Ibid., 18.
8. Ibid., 19.
9. Ibid., 20.
10. Ibid., 56–62.
11. Ibid., 192.
12. Ibid., 61.
13. Ibid., 330–36.
14. Ibid., 333.
15. Roger L. Gould, *Transformations* (New York: Simon and Schuster, 1978), 14.
16. Ibid., 18.
17. Ibid., 24.
18. Ibid., 25.
19. Carol Gilligan, "Adult Development and Women's Development: Arrangements for a Marriage," in *Women in the Middle Years*, ed. Janet Zollinger Giele (New York: John Wiley and Sons, 1982), 89.

20. Levinson et al., *Seasons of a Man's Life*, 8.

21. Gilligan, "Adult Development and Women's Development," 106.

22. D. G. Maguigan, cited in Janet Zollinger Giele, "Women in Adulthood: Unanswered Questions," in *Women in the Middle Years*, ed. Janet Zollinger Giele (New York: John Wiley and Sons, 1982), 11.

23. Carol Gilligan, *In a Different Voice: Psychological Theory and Women's Development* (Cambridge: Harvard University Press, 1982).

24. Janet Zollinger Giele, "Women in Adulthood: Unanswered Questions," 10.

25. Ruthellen Josselson, *Finding Herself: Pathways to Identity Development in Women* (San Francisco: Jossey-Bass, 1987), 23.

26. Ibid., 168.

27. Ibid., 27.

28. Iris Sangiuliano, *In Her Time* (New York: Morrow, 1978), 20.

29. Ibid., 324.

30. Ibid., 158–60.

31. Daniel Goleman, Paul Kaufman, and Michael Ray, *The Creative Spirit* (New York: Dutton, 1992).

32. Joanne F. Vickers and Barbara L. Thomas, *No More Frogs, No More Princes: Women Making Creative Choices at Midlife* (Freedom, Calif.: Crossing Press, 1993), 7.

33. Ibid., 8.

34. Maggie Scarf, *Unfinished Business: Pressure Points in the Lives of Women* (New York: Doubleday, 1980), 6–7.

35. John Franklin Roschen, *Baby Boomers Face Midlife: Implications for Faith Communities in the Nineties and Beyond* (Minneapolis: Adult Faith Resources, 1991), 3.

36. Ibid., 17.

37. Ross Goldstein with Diana Landau, *Fortysomething* (Los Angeles: Jeremy P. Tarcher, 1990), 20.

38. Cheryl Merser, *"Grown Ups": A Generation in Search of Adulthood* (New York: G. P. Putnam's Sons, 1987), 22–23.

39. Ibid., 179.

40. Gail Sheehy, *New Passages: Mapping Your Life Across Time* (New York: Random House, 1995).

41. Ibid., 3–20.

42. Ibid., 138–49.

43. *Life Insurance Fact Book* (Washington D.C.: American Council of Life Insurance, 1994).

44. American Board of Family Practice, *Perspectives on Middle Ages: The Vintage Years* (Lexington, Ky.: American Board of Family Practice, 1990), 23.

45. Karen Blaker, *Celebrating Fifty* (Chicago: Contemporary Books, 1990), 2.

46. Ibid., 16.

47. Lillian E. Troll, "Family Life in Middle and Old Age: The Generation Gap," in *Middle and Late Life Transitions: The Annals of the American Academy of Political and Social Science* 464 (November 1982): 41 (Beverly Hills: Sage Publications).

48. Giele, "Women in Adulthood," 8.

49. William Bridges, *Transitions* (Reading, Mass.: Addison-Wesley, 1980), 24.

50. Ibid., 42ff.

51. Anne Brennan and Janice Brewi, *Mid-Life Directions* (New York: Paulist Press, 1985), 20.

52. Ibid., 48.

2. Health Management

1. Richard Benyo and Rhonda Provost, *Feeling Fit in Your 40's* (New York: Atheneum, 1987), 11.

2. *Bostonia*, 52, no. 1 (winter 1978), published by the Office of Public Relations of Boston University. This research was done on males. I could not find exact parallel information for females, but the trends would certainly be parallel.

3. Benyo and Provost, *Feeling Fit in Your 40's*, 6–8; Bernard A. Eskin and Lynne S. Dumas, *Midlife Can Wait: How to Stay Young and Healthy after 35* (New York: Ballantine Books, 1995), 37.

4. Harris H. McIlwain, Lori F. Steinmeyer, Debra Fulghum Bruce, R. E. Fulghum, and Robert G. Bruce Jr. *The 50+ Wellness Program* (New York: John Wiley and Sons, 1990), 51.

5. Ibid., 51–52.

6. Ibid., 11–24.

7. Gail Sheehy, *The Silent Passage: Menopause* (New York: Random House, 1991).

8. Tom Monte, *Staying Young: How to Prevent, Slow, or Reverse More Than 60 Signs of Aging* (Emmaus, Pa.: Rodale Press, 1994), 3–5.

9. Benyo and Provost, *Feeling Fit in Your 40's*, 63.

10. Monte, *Staying Young*, 4–10.

11. Benyo and Provost, *Feeling Fit in Your 40's*, 115–16.

12. Robert L. Rowan, *How to Control High Blood Pressure Without Drugs* (New York: Charles Scribner's Sons, 1986), 29.

13. Jane E. Brody, "China's Blockbuster Diet Study," *Saturday Evening Post*, October 1990, 30.

14. Ibid., 32.

15. Cory SerVaas, "Diets That Protected Against Cancers in China," *Saturday Evening Post*, October 1990, 27–28.

16. Monte, *Staying Young*, 154.

17. Benyo and Provost, *Feeling Fit in Your 40's*, 31–36.

18. Brody, "China's Blockbuster Diet Study," 30.

19. McIlwain et al., *The 50+ Wellness Program*, 53.

20. Benyo and Provost, *Feeling Fit in Your 40's*, 39–40.

21. Monte, *Staying Young*, 128–30.

22. *Bostonia*, 15.

23. Benyo and Provost, *Feeling Fit in Your 40's*, 149–89.

24. Bernie S. Siegel, *Love, Medicine, and Miracles* (New York: Harper and Row, 1986), 145.

25. Norman Cousins, "The Laughter Prescription," *Saturday Evening Post*, October 1990, 39.

26. Ibid., 34.

27. Ibid., 39.

28. Monte, *Staying Young*, 312–17.

29. Lloyd Ogilvie, *Making Stress Work for You* (Waco, Tex.: Word Books, 1984), 68.

30. Ibid.

31. Ibid., 202–3.

32. Siegel, *Love, Medicine, and Miracles*, 203–4.

33. Bruce Larson, *There's a Lot More to Health Than Not Being Sick* (Waco, Tex.: Word Books, 1981), 138–39.

34. Siegel, *Love, Medicine, and Miracles*, 105–8.

35. Larson, *There's a Lot More to Health*, 46–47.

36. Ibid., 136.

3. Career Decisions

1. Carole Hyatt, *Shifting Gears* (New York: Simon and Schuster, 1990), 23.

2. Ibid., 30.

3. Jack Falvey, *What's Next? Career Strategies after 35* (Charlotte, N.C.: Williamson Publishing, 1987), 26.

4. Hyatt, *Shifting Gears*, 25–34.

5. Ibid., 24.

6. Ibid., 22–23.

7. Richard Nelson Bolles, *What Color Is Your Parachute?* (Berkeley, Calif.: Ten Speed Press, 1995), iii.

8. Samuel N. Ray, *Job Hunting after 50* (New York: John Wiley and Sons, 1991), 28–33.

9. Jo Dana, *It's Never Too Late to Start Over* (Briarwood, N.Y.: Palomino Press, 1983), 9.

10. Stephen Strasser and John Sena, *Transitions: Successful Strategies from Mid-Career to Retirement* (Hawthorne, N.J.: The Career Press, 1990), 111.

11. Ibid., 109–13.

12. Dave Barry, *Dave Barry Turns 40* (New York: Fawcett Columbine, 1990), 77-79.

13. Tom Jackson, *Not Just Another Job* [New York: Times Books (Random House), 1992], 46.

14. Ibid., 84–85.

15. Carole Hyatt, *Shifting Gears* (New York: Simon and Schuster, 1990), 47.

16. Ibid., 48.

17. Ibid., 56.

18. Ibid., 62–63.

19. Ibid., 69.

20. Ibid., 77.

21. Frederick Buechner, *Wishful Thinking: A Theological ABC* (New York: Harper and Row, 1979), 95.

22. Richard Nelson Bolles, *The Three Boxes of Life and How to Get Out of Them* (Berkeley: Ten Speed Press, 1978), 138–39.

23. John L. Holland, *Making Vocational Choices* (Englewood Cliffs: Prentice-Hall, Inc., 1985); David Srebalus, "Vocational Choice: John

Holland's Theory," in *The Encyclopedia of Career Change and Work Issues*, ed. Lawrence K. Jones (Phoenix: Oryx Press, 1992), 319–21.

24. Bolles, *What Color Is Your Parachute?*, 117.

25. Tom Jackson, *Not Just Another Job* [New York: Times Books (Random House), 1992], 39, 110, 125–49.

26. Strasser and Sena, *Transitions*, 127.

27. Bolles, *The Three Boxes of Life*

28. Viktor Frankl, *The Will to Meaning* (New York: New American Library, 1969), 69–71.

29. Strasser and Sena, *Transitions*, 172–74.

30. John S. Morgan, *Getting a Job after 50* (Princeton, N.J.: Petrocelli Books, 1987), 6.

31. Falvey, *What's Next?*, 172.

32. Ray, *Job Hunting after 50*, 7– 8.

33. Ibid., xi.

34. Morgan, *Getting a Job after 50*, 10.

35. Strasser and Sena, *Transitions*, 163–65.

36. Ray, *Job Hunting after 50*, 59.

4. Marriage

1. Eda LeShan, *The Wonderful Crisis of Middle Age* (New York: David McKay, Co., Inc., Warner Books Edition, 1973), 81.

2. Sonya Rhodes with Susan Schneider, *Second Honeymoon: A Pioneering Guide for Reviving the Mid-Life Marriage* (New York: Morrow, 1992), 78.

3. Bill Cosby, *Love and Marriage* (New York: Bantam Books, 1989, 1990), 227–29.

4. Jane Porcino, *Growing Older, Getting Better* (New York: Continuum, 1983, 1991), 197.

5. Rhodes, *Second Honeymoon*, 197.

6. Ross Goldstein, *Fortysomething* (Los Angeles: Jeremy P. Tarcher, 1990), 175–76.

7. Barbara Fried, *The Middle-Age Crisis* (New York: Harper and Row, 1967), 102.

8. Rhodes, *Second Honeymoon*, 60.

9. Ibid., 82, 252–53.

10. Richard P. Olson and Joe H. Leonard Jr., *Ministry with Families in Flux* (Louisville: Westminster John Knox Press, 1990), 5.
11. Robert Lee and Marjorie Casebier, *The Spouse Gap* (Nashville: Abingdon Press, 1971), 82–83.
12. Goldstein, *Fortysomething*, 182.
13. Cosby, *Love and Marriage*, 206–8.
14. Goldstein, *Fortysomething*, 183–85.
15. William Bridges, *Transitions* (Reading, Mass.: Addison-Wesley, 1980), 61.
16. Erma Bombeck, *Aunt Erma's Cope Book* (New York: McGraw-Hill, 1979), 18–19.
17. Rhodes, *Second Honeymoon*, 251.
18. Ibid., 31–138.
19. Ibid., 28.
20. Bridges, *Transitions*, 89–150.
21. Rhodes, *Second Honeymoon*, 15–16.
22. Further information may be obtained by writing to Marriage Enrichment, P.O. Box 10596, Winston-Salem, NC 27103, or to United Marriage Encounter, P.O. Box 209, Muscatine, IA 52761.
23. Ibid., 207.
24. Warren Lane Molton, *Friends, Partners, and Lovers* (Valley Forge, Pa.: Judson Press, 1995), 78.
25. Goldstein, *Fortysomething*, 192.

5. Singleness and Remarriage

1. Carolyn A. Koons and Michael J. Anthony, *Single Adult Passages: Uncharted Territories* (Grand Rapids, Mich.: Baker Book House, 1991), 49–51, 59.
2. Porcino, *Growing Older, Getting Better*, 27–29.
3. Koons and Anthony, *Single Adult Passages*, 27.
4. John R. Landgraf, *Singling: A New Way to Live the Single Life* (Louisville: Westminster John Knox, 1990), 45–51.
5. Porcino, *Growing Older, Getting Better*, 42.
6. Koons and Anthony, *Single Adult Passages*, 92.
7. Landgraf, *Singling*, 59.
8. Ibid., 57–66.

9. J. Smoke, *Living Beyond Divorce—The Possibilities of Remarriage* (Eugene, Oreg.: Harvest House, 1984).

10. Porcino, *Growing Older, Getting Better*, 41.

11. Koons and Anthony, *Single Adult Passages*, 60.

12. James J. Young, *Divorcing, Believing, Belonging* (New York: Paulist Press, 1984), 35.

13. Eda LeShan, *Oh, to Be 50 Again!* (New York: Times Books, 1986), 314, 318.

14. Young, *Divorcing, Believing, Belonging*, 36.

15. Koons and Anthony, *Single Adult Passages*, 123.

16. Landgraf, *Singling*, 160–69.

17. *Source Book of Health Insurance Data* (Washington, D.C.: Health Insurance Association of American, 1995), 149.

18. Ibid., chap. 10.

19. Koons and Anthony, *Single Adult Passages*, 67.

20. Landgraf, *Singling*, 16–18.

21. Richard P. Olson and Joe H. Leonard, *A New Day for Family Ministry* (Bethesda, Md.: Albin Institute, 1996).

22. Rodney Clapp, *Families at the Crossroads* (Downers Grove, Ill.: Intervarsity Press, 1983), 113.

23. Koons and Anthony, *Single Adult Passages*, 78–79.

24. Young, *Divorcing, Believing, Belonging*, 74.

25. Emily B. Visher and John S. Visher, *Stepfamilies: A Guide to Working with Stepparents and Stepchildren* (New York: Brunner/Mazel, 1988), 10.

26. Florence W. Kaslow and Lita Linzer Schwartz, *The Dynamics of Divorce: A Life Cycle Perspective* (New York: Brunner/Mazel Publishers, 1987), 348.

27. Porcino, *Growing Older, Getting Better*, 60.

28. Richard P. Olson and Carole Della Pia-Terry, *Help for Remarried Couples and Families* (Valley Forge, Pa.: Judson Press, 1984), 135–39.

6. Being Parents

1. Andrew L. Yarrow, *Latecomers: Children of Parents Over 35* (New York: Free Press, 1991), 4.

2. Ibid., 175.

3. Ibid., 103–11.

4. Ibid., 18.

5. Ibid., 112–27.

6. Ibid., 188.

7. Ibid., 214–22.

8. Barbara M. Newman and Philip R. Newman, *Development through Life: A Psychosocial Approach* (Homewood, Ill.: Dorsey Press, 1979), 268–85.

9. Ibid., 312–25.

10. Quentin F. Schenk and Emmy Lou Schenk, *Pulling Up Roots* (Englewood Cliffs, N.J.: Prentice-Hall, 1978), 5.

11. Levinson et al., *Seasons of a Man's Life*, 56–62.

12. Zenith Henkin Gross, *And You Thought It Was All Over!* (New York: St. Martin's/Marek, 1985), xiii.

13. Karen Levin Coburn and Madge Lawrence Treeger, *Letting Go: A Parents' Guide to Today's College Experience* (Bethesda, Md.: Adler and Adler, 1988), 124.

14. Ibid., 128–29.

15. Luther B. Otto, *How to Help Your Child Choose a Career* (New York: M. Evans and Company, 1984), 28.

16. Ibid., 21, 53–60.

17. Gross, *And You Thought It Was All Over!*, 70.

18. Ibid., 69–93.

19. Richard P. Olson and Helen E. Froyd, *Discoveries: Expanding Your Child's Vocational Horizon* (Cleveland: United Church Press, 1995).

20. Jean Davies Okimoto and Phyllis Jackson Stegall, *Boomerang Kids: How to Live with Adult Children Who Return Home* (Boston: Little, Brown, 1987), 5.

21. Gross, *And You Thought It Was All Over!*, 216.

22. Okimoto and Stegall, *Boomerang Kids*, 14.

23. Gross, *And You Thought It Was All Over!*, 221–22; Okimoto and Stegall, *Boomerang Kids*, 128–46.

24. Okimoto and Stegall, *Boomerang Kids*, 93.

25. Ibid., 62.

26. Ibid., 65.

27. Gross, *And You Thought It Was All Over!*, 171.

28. Ibid., 172.

29. Ibid., 202.

7. Caring for Our Parents

1. Helene MacLean, *Caring For Your Parents* (Garden City, N.Y.: Doubleday, 1987), 26.
2. Ibid., 26–55.
3. Ibid., 26.
4. Judah L. Ronch, *Alzheimer's Disease: A Practical Guide for Those Who Help Others* (New York: Continuum, 1989), 175–76.
5. Ibid., 171–74.
6. Ibid., 20–21.
7. Ibid., 35.
8. Mark A. Edinberg, *Talking With Your Aging Parents* (Boston: Shambhala, 1987), 14–15.
9. Ibid., 2–3.
10. Tom Koch, *Mirrored Lives: Aging Children and Elderly Parents* (New York: Praeger, 1990), 18.
11. Ibid., 187.
12. Ibid., 189–99.
13. Ibid., 3.
14. Henri J. M. Nouwen and Walter J. Gaffney, *Aging: The Fulfillment of Life* (Garden City, N.Y.: Image Books, 1976), 154.
15. Barbara Silverstone and Helen Kandel Hyman, *You and Your Aging Parents* (New York: Pantheon Books, 1976), 11.

8. Facing Death in Myself and Those I Love

1. Elizabeth Kubler-Ross, *On Death and Dying* (New York: Macmillan, 1969), 141.
2. Ibid., 39.
3. Kenneth R. Mitchell and Herbert Anderson, *All Our Losses, All Our Griefs* (Philadelphia: Westminster Press, 1983), 36.
4. Ibid., 37–38.
5. Ibid., 40.
6. Ibid., 41.
7. Ibid., 42.
8. Elizabeth Kubler-Ross, *Death, the Final Stage of Growth* (Englewood Cliffs, N.J.: Prentice-Hall, 1975), 10.
9. Ibid., 161.
10. Ibid.

11. M. Scott Peck, *Further Along the Road Less Traveled* (New York: Simon and Schuster, 1993), 63.
12. Derek Humphry, *Final Exit: The Practicalities of Self-Deliverance and Assisted Suicide for the Dying* (Eugene, Oreg.: The Hemlock Society, 1991), 18.
13. Ibid., 20–21.
14. Siegel, *Love, Medicine, and Miracles*, 207.
15. Ruth Jean Loewinsohn, *Survival Handbook for Widows* (Chicago: Follett Publishing, 1979), 69–77.
16. Mitchell and Anderson, *All Our Losses, All Our Griefs*, 62–85.
17. Robert Jay Lifton and Eric Olson, *Living and Dying* (New York: Praeger Publishers, 1974), 77.
18. Ibid., 77.
19. Kubler-Ross, *Death, the Final Stage of Growth*, 36–37.
20. Jim Conway, *Men in Mid Life Crisis* (Elgin, Ill.: David C. Cook, 1978), 270.
21. Raymond A. Moody Jr., *Life after Life* (New York: Bantam Books, 1976), 92–93.
22. William J. Worden and William Proctor, *Personal Death Awareness* (Englewood Cliffs, N.J.: Prentice-Hall, 1976), 69.
23. Siegel, *Love, Medicine, and Miracles*, 24–25.

9. Exploring Myself and My Faith

1. Patrick L. Carroll, S.J., and Katherine Marie Dyckman, *Chaos or Creation: Spirituality in Mid-Life* (Mahwah, N.J.: Paulist Press, 1986), 26.
2. Janice Brewi and Anne Brennan, *Midlife: Psychological and Spiritual Perspectives* (New York: Crossroad, 1982), 47, 50.
3. Ibid., 46.
4. Ibid., 4.
5. Ibid., 62.
6. Evelyn Eaton Whitehead and James D. Whitehead, *Seasons of Strength: New Visions of Christian Maturing* (New York: Doubleday, 1984), 23.
7. Ibid., 23–28.
8. Ibid., 35.
9. Dorothy Parker, *The Portable Dorothy Parker* (New York: Viking Press, 1954).

10. M. Scott Peck, *The Road Less Traveled* (New York: Simon and Schuster, 1978), 15.

11. Roschen, *Baby Boomers Face Midlife*, 88.

12. Ibid., 89–90, 15–44.

13. Kenneth Stokes, *Faith Is a Verb* (Mystic, Conn.: Twenty-Third Publications, 1989), 4–5.

14. Ibid., 5.

15. Ibid., 5.

16. John Westerhoff, *Will Our Children Have Faith?* (New York: Seabury Press, 1976), 96.

17. Stokes, *Faith Is a Verb*, 14.

18. Ibid., 12.

19. Westerhoff, *Will Our Children*, 89–99.

20. Charles McCullough, *Head of Heaven, Feet of Clay* (Cleveland: The Pilgrim Press, 1981), 6.

21. James W. Fowler, *Stages of Faith* (San Francisco: Harper and Row, 1981), 201.

22. James Fowler and Sam Keen, *Life Maps: Conversations on the Journey of Faith* (Waco, Tex.: Word Books, 1978), 120.

23. Ibid.; Sam Keen, *The Passionate Life: Stages of Loving* (New York: Harper and Row, 1983).

24. Stokes, *Faith Is a Verb*; McCullough, *Head of Heaven, Feet of Clay*; Keen, *The Passionate Life: Stages of Loving*.

25. Stokes, *Faith Is a Verb*, 1.

26. Ibid., 27.

27. Leslie Weatherhead, *The Christian Agnostic* (Nashville: Abingdon, 1965), 15.

28. Many of the issues discussed in this chapter were previously explored in slightly different form in the following: Richard P. Olson, "Personal Becoming and Life Stages," *Baptist Leader* 46, no. 6 (Valley Forge, Pa.: Judson Press), September 1984.

29. Wade Clark Roof et al., *A Generation of Seekers: The Spiritual Journeys of the Baby Boom Generation* (San Francisco: Harper, 1993), 30–31, 59–65.

30. Stokes, *Faith Is a Verb*, 69.

31. Roschen, *Baby Boomers Face Midlife*, 61–62.

32. Roof, *A Generation of Seekers:*, 64–65.

33. Peck, *The Road Less Traveled*, 11.

34. Howard Clinebell, *Growth Counseling* (Nashville: Abingdon, 1979), 19.

35. Carroll and Dyckman, *Chaos or Creation*, 48, 63–64.

36. Kathleen Fischer, *Autumn Gospel: Women in the Second Half of Life* (New York: Paulist Press, 1995), 45.

10. Credo of a Midlife Christian

1. Janice Brewi and Anne Brennan, *Celebrate Mid-Life: Jungian Archetypes and Mid-Life Spirituality* (New York: Crossroad, 1990), 12.

2. David J. Maitland, *Looking Both Ways: A Theology for Mid-Life* (Atlanta: John Knox Press, 1985), 147.

3. Ibid., 148–49.

4. Craig Kennet Miller, *Baby Boomer Spirituality: Ten Essential Values of a Generation* (Nashville: Discipleship Resources, 1992), 61.

5. Ibid., 60.

6. Ibid., 69.

7. Ibid., 72.

8. Ibid., 82.

9. Ibid., 83.

10. John Powell, *He Touched Me: My Pilgrimage of Prayer* (Niles, Ill.: Argus Communications, 1974), 70.

11. Eugene C. Bianchi, *Aging as a Spiritual Journey* (New York: Crossroad, 1989), 47.

12. Ibid.

13. Miller, *Baby Boomer Spirituality*, 119–30.

14. Fischer, *Autumn Gospel*.

15. Brennan and Brewi, *Mid-Life Directions*, 165.

16. Ibid., 167–68.

17. Ibid., 118–21.

18. Ibid., 145.

19. Robert P. Buford, *Halftime: Changing Your Game Plan from Success to Significance* (Grand Rapids, Mich.: Zondervan Publishing House, 1994), 16–24.

20. William Barclay, *The Gospel of John* (Edinburgh: The Saint Andrew Press, 1956), 113–14.

21. Sangiuliano, *In Her Time*, 19.

22. Sheehy, *New Passages*, xiii.

23. Brewi and Brennan, *Celebrate Mid-Life*, 33.
24. Roschen, *Baby Boomers Face Midlife*, 37.
25. Bianchi, *Aging as a Spiritual Journey*, 8.
26. Miller, *Baby Boomer Spirituality*, 86.

Index